Teaching Inpatient Medicine

T0331995

Teaching Inpatient Medicine

*Connecting, Coaching &
Communicating in the Hospital*

Second Edition

Nathan Houchens, MD
Molly Harrod, PhD
Sanjay Saint, MD, MPH

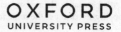

OXFORD
UNIVERSITY PRESS

Oxford University Press is a department of the University of Oxford. It furthers
the University's objective of excellence in research, scholarship, and education
by publishing worldwide. Oxford is a registered trade mark of Oxford University
Press in the UK and certain other countries.

Published in the United States of America by Oxford University Press
198 Madison Avenue, New York, NY 10016, United States of America.

Library of Congress Cataloging-in-Publication Data
Names: Harrod, Molly, author. | Houchens, Nathan, author. | Saint, Sanjay, author.
Title: Teaching inpatient medicine : connecting, coaching & communicating in the
hospital / Nathan Houchens, Molly Harrod, Sanjay Saint.
Description: Second edition. | New York, NY : Oxford University Press, 2023. |
Molly Harrod's name appears first in the previous edition. |
Includes bibliographical references and index.
Identifiers: LCCN 2022042493 (print) | LCCN 2022042494 (ebook) |
ISBN 9780197639023 (paperback) | ISBN 9780197639047 (epub) |
ISBN 9780197639054
Subjects: MESH: Education, Medical | Internship and Residency—standards |
Hospital Medicine—education | Group Processes
Classification: LCC R737 (print) | LCC R737 (ebook) | NLM W 18 |
DDC 610.71/1—dc23/eng/20230103
LC record available at https://lccn.loc.gov/2022042493
LC ebook record available at https://lccn.loc.gov/2022042494

DOI: 10.1093/oso/9780197639023.001.0001

Printed by Marquis, Canada

To all those patients and colleagues who have graciously offered the gift of a glimpse into their lives.
—Nathan Houchens

To all the great teachers and those in the making.
—Molly Harrod

To the 18 superb attending physicians who allowed us to learn so much from them.
—Sanjay Saint

Contents

Preface

Our book—*Teaching Inpatient Medicine: Connecting, Coaching & Communicating in the Hospital, Second Edition*—is aimed at those who want to become better inpatient teaching attending physicians. Medical education on the wards must, increasingly, be high-yield, given resident work duty restrictions and the imperative to deliver high-quality, efficient care despite the strain that the COVID-19 pandemic has placed on healthcare workers. This educational responsibility falls on the shoulders of the attendings: supervising physicians who have been educated themselves in the system, few of whom have had any formal training in the art of teaching.

Attendings must teach more than the scientific knowledge and technical skills necessary to deliver quality care. Physicians-in-training must learn how to communicate with patients, family members, and other healthcare providers; they must learn professionalism, time management, and how to be independent while also serving as an active member of the team. To provide high quality and value to patients, we must ensure that physicians-in-training receive high quality and value in their clinical education. The shift from a physician-centric model of care to a relationship-centered model requires physicians to communicate and interact with individuals they may not have collaborated with in the past. Attending physicians, who may have been educated under the previous model, now must teach the next generation how to deliver care that is inter-disciplinary, team-based, and patient-centered.

The successful attending physician will also have constraints on time. Not only are they responsible for the medical team but, first and foremost, for patient care. Attendings in the 21st century care for more complex patients, have more interactions with other healthcare providers in the hospital (e.g., consulting physicians, radiologists, pharmacists, social workers, discharge planners), and spend more time on documentation—not to mention the continued responsibilities of the work they do when not attending on the hospital wards.

Additionally, as we discuss in this new edition, the myriad attending responsibilities are often met with complex social and cultural challenges surrounding gender, race, color, and ethnicity. Research has been conducted that reveals various strategies that female and underrepresented minority teaching attendings use to navigate these challenges in clinical environments like the hospital wards. Amid these challenges, attendings are also poised to play key roles as mentors, guiding and walking alongside mentees and peers. The ways that stellar teaching physicians both provide and receive mentorship will also be highlighted in this book, along with practical examples.

Despite all the competing and difficult aspects of clinical training, this system of clinical medical education remains the cornerstone of preparing new generations of physicians. As might be expected, the quality of teaching that attendings provide is varied. What is it that makes one more effective than another? We believe there are opportunities to learn from those who are considered outstanding teachers. By studying how highly regarded attendings manage the complexity of the wards, both junior and more established attendings can elevate their own skills.

While other research has focused on how clinical teachers approach the learning environment and what they do within those boundaries, these studies tend to focus on only one perspective (students or teachers). They often do not take into account multiple perspectives on the same team or in the same study (e.g., focus is on medical students or interns), nor do they look at the roles that other healthcare workers and patients play in the learning process. To understand teaching as a lifelong process, we must go beyond asking what personal attributes an attending should have and instead ask what type of learning environment the best attendings create and how they manage and change this environment as different emphases on patient care emerge. In our first edition, we turned to the wards to understand how the next generation of physicians was learning to care for patients, to examine the environments great teaching attendings created, and to elucidate methods to teach multilevel learners to provide exceptional care. For this edition, we return to the wards, in part with the same questions, while also learning from the techniques and strategies of a more diverse group of teaching physicians. We return, in part, to understand the sometimes invisible challenges they face, how they navigate biases based on their intersecting identities, how they teach learners to compassionately communicate with patients, and how they continue educating in the face of crises. We sought to use our research findings to help guide other attendings who are looking for ways to improve their approach to teaching.

This book is the work of two internal medicine attending physicians who have had a long-standing interest in medical education, and a medical anthropologist with expertise in using qualitative techniques in healthcare settings. We purposely chose to write using a conversational style, rich in practice-based anecdotes. While the primary audience is the teaching attending physician who wishes to improve their skills (ranging from the recent graduate to the attending with decades of experience), medical educators, inpatient directors, and physicians-in-training may also find our results and recommendations useful.

Many people helped bring this book to fruition. First and foremost, we would like to thank the attendings and their teams (both current and former) who welcomed us into a "day in their life" and shared with us their time, knowledge, thoughts, and experiences. It goes without saying that this book would not have been possible without all of you. Second, a huge thank you to Karen E. Fowler who planned, organized, and kept the research on schedule. Third, thank you to Rachel Ehrlinger who managed and coordinated all aspects of production of this edition of the book. Fourth, profound thanks to Martha Quinn for her eminent assistance in data collection and careful analysis. Fifth, deep appreciation to Robert Stock for his contributions to the first edition. And, finally, to our families, who saw us off for each site visit, fully supportive of the work we were doing.

We hope you enjoy reading the book as much as we have enjoyed writing it.

Nathan Houchens, MD
Molly Harrod, PhD
Sanjay Saint, MD, MPH

About the Authors

Nathan Houchens, MD, FHM, FACP, is the Associate Chief of Medicine at the VA Ann Arbor Healthcare System, an Associate Professor of Internal Medicine at the University of Michigan, and an Assistant Program Director for the Internal Medicine Residency at the University of Michigan. His scholarly work focuses on effective teaching in hospital environments, communication and the patient–physician relationship, and clinical reasoning and problem-solving. He is a National Correspondent for the *Journal of Hospital Medicine* and a regular contributor to *BMJ Quality & Safety*. He received his Medical Doctorate from the University of Illinois at Chicago College of Medicine and completed a medical residency and chief residency at the University of Michigan. He is the recipient of multiple teaching awards, including the Special Recognition for Contributions to the Medical Student Teaching Program and the Richard D. Judge Award for Excellence in Medical Student Teaching, both from the University of Michigan.

Molly Harrod, PhD, is a medical anthropologist and Health Services Researcher with the VA Ann Arbor Center for Clinical Management Research. She was the lead author on the first edition of *Teaching Inpatient Medicine*. She has been involved in numerous qualitative and mixed-methods studies focusing on topics such as clinician communication and teamwork, provider training and decision-making, behavior change, patient safety, and implementation science. She has trained other health researchers in qualitative methods including semi-structured interviewing and the use of observation in research.

Sanjay Saint, MD, MPH, MACP, is the Chief of Medicine at the VA Ann Arbor Healthcare System, the George Dock Professor of

Internal Medicine at the University of Michigan, and the Director of the VA/University of Michigan Patient Safety Enhancement Program. His scholarly work focuses on enhancing patient safety, clinical decision-making, and medical education. He has authored more than 400 peer-reviewed papers and co-authored several books published by Oxford University Press, including *Preventing Hospital Infections, Teaching Inpatient Medicine: What Every Physician Needs to Know,* and *The Saint-Chopra Guide to Inpatient Medicine* (4th edition). He has also co-authored two books published by the University of Michigan: *Thirty Rules for Healthcare Leaders* and *The Mentoring Guide: Helping Mentors and Mentees Succeed.* He is a special correspondent to the *New England Journal of Medicine,* an editorial board member of *BMJ Quality and Safety,* an elected member of the American Society for Clinical Investigation and the Association of American Physicians, and an international honorary fellow of the Royal College of Physicians (FRCP), and he received Mastership in the American College of Physicians (MACP). He received his Medical Doctorate from the University of California, Los Angeles; completed a medical residency and chief residency at the University of California, San Francisco; and obtained a Master's in Public Health (as a Robert Wood Johnson Clinical Scholar) from the University of Washington, Seattle. He has been a visiting professor at more than 100 universities and hospitals in the United States, Europe, and Asia.

1
Teaching Medicine

*Leadership is about making others better as a result of your
presence and making sure that impact lasts in your absence.*

—Sheryl Sandberg

At the beginning of a small-group teaching session, the teaching
attending physician asked all team members to draw flow-volume
curves that would be representative of normal physiology and different disease states. The attending mentioned to the senior medical resident, "This is important since it will definitely show up on
your board examination." As the learners worked to map out the
drawings, the attending recognized the difficulty of the request and
instead of being demeaning, was encouraging in her approach: "If
you have the normal curve down, congratulate yourself." This positive reinforcement helped team members bolster their confidence
before undertaking increasingly difficult steps.

As the session went on, she posed questions to individuals and
the group that were aimed at various levels of learner achievement: "What symptoms will a patient with chronic obstructive pulmonary disease report? What is your first-line treatment? How can
you determine if the patient responds to bronchodilator therapy?
When would you give antibiotics for an acute exacerbation?" When
learners responded correctly, the attending would point at the
learner, say their name, and exclaim, "Yes, excellent!"

The attending demonstrated humility and admitted gaps in
her own knowledge: "Roflumilast was something new for me that

Teaching Inpatient Medicine. Second Edition. Nathan Houchens, Molly Harrod, and Sanjay Saint,
Oxford University Press. © Nathan Houchens, Molly Harrod, and Sanjay Saint 2023.
DOI: 10.1093/oso/9780197639023.003.0001

I encountered in my own studying. I didn't know *what* that was." In closing the session, the attending asked a blunt question: "When reviewing pulmonary function tests, how many of you pull up the actual report yourselves and how many just read the interpretation?" When several team members candidly admitted that they only rely on the pulmonologist's interpretation, the attending did not express disappointment or serve out admonishments. Rather, she inspired her learners with why the teaching session was important to their future careers: "I want to get it such that you feel comfortable reading the primary study results."

This real scenario is but one example of many similar teaching sessions occurring in hospitals and healthcare systems across the country in which the attending physician commits themselves to creating a safe, supportive, inclusive learning environment that is tailored to individual learners. Yet this style requires much energy and dedicated effort, particularly given the number of challenges that have arisen in modern healthcare and that threaten effective teaching in medicine.

Challenges Abound

Gradually, and then in a rush over the past few decades, the world of medicine and hospitals, in particular, have undergone seismic changes. Today's attendings and learners are part of a very different and far more complex and demanding hospital environment. Medical education has perhaps never been so challenging.

Medical schools in the United States now graduate some 20,000 students a year, and most of them will continue their medical education at one of the more than 1,000 teaching hospitals.[1,2] These institutions, although just 5% of all hospitals, provide 98% of the nation's 41 comprehensive cancer centers, 71% of all level-one trauma centers, 69% of all burn unit beds, and 63% of pediatric intensive care units.[3] They are intense, varied environments. There, along with graduates of international medical schools, learners will be entrusted to a series of attending physicians who may have had little or no training in the art and theory of teaching and who must navigate storms of pressures and distractions, from inside and out.

Advances in medical knowledge and technology have made it nearly impossible for any single physician to handle a patient's care. Attendings now function as part of a large team that includes patients, family members, and surrogate decision-makers as partners in care, as well as an interdisciplinary group of nurses, technicians, pharmacists, social workers, physical and occupational therapists, dieticians, interpreters, radiologists, and other specialists, to name a few. A 2007 study from New Zealand noted that the number of health professionals who interact with a single hospitalized medical patient was 17 or more and, with a single hospitalized surgical patient, 26 or more.[4]

Effective teamwork calls for personal qualities such as empathy and communication, skills that were not especially emphasized among attendings in previous generations. Moreover, the historic physician-centered model of hospital care has evolved to a patient-centered or relationship-centered model. Hospitals list patient satisfaction alongside high-quality healthcare as one of their primary goals, and literature has shown links connecting a good healthcare experience to patient safety and important health outcomes, such as better adherence to medication, treatment plans, and preventive care; fewer medical errors; and lower healthcare utilization.[5] When talking with patients and their families, attendings and learners collaborate and engage in shared decision-making, routinely incorporating patients' views and goals into treatment decisions.

The time pressure on today's attending physicians is unprecedented. As in years past, they must care for their own patients in addition to their teaching duties and any other necessary work when not attending on the wards, such as administrative or research responsibilities. But now, as the general population has aged, attendings are treating patients with far more complex problems—and this at a time when hospitals are discharging patients sooner than ever before. Attendings and their teams have less time to spend with individual patients who, in the past, might have stayed in the hospital for several weeks. This gave learners more time to become familiar with the medical issues and treatment outcomes, but these patients now leave in a matter of days. The number of pharmaceutical drugs continues to climb, with more than 20,000 prescription drug products approved for marketing.[6] The time spent in bedside rounding—an indispensable element of clinical education—has shrunk, while the hours devoted to billing and coding, administrative matters, and work within the electronic medical record have multiplied.

As a demonstration of how administrative activities can interrupt learning: when we were accompanying one attending on rounds, an intern had to step away several times to answer a page about a patient transfer. When team members get pulled away to deal with "administrative stuff," the attending said, "It drives me nuts!"

In an effort to reduce medical errors by exhausted learners, the maximum amount of time resident physicians could spend on patient care in the hospital per work week was limited to 80 hours in 2003, and a single shift cap of 16 hours for interns was instituted in 2011.[7] These changes have substantially increased the time pressure on both attendings and learners. Learners now have fewer hours in which to accomplish the same workload—and attendings have less time to facilitate learning an increasingly complex body of medical knowledge. Compression of learners' hours has also inspired frequent schedule adjustments. As a result, the members of an attending's team may vary from day to day, thus depriving them of the essential experience of caring for a single group of patients, interrupting the sense of camaraderie, and breaking the continuity of the attending's instruction.

Just as attending physicians must use their time wisely to achieve their goals, they also face a number of internal and external disruptions to their ability to teach effectively. Attendings often encounter a myriad of competing demands among their personal and professional lives. They must balance the autonomy of learners, their clinical education, and the safety and healthcare experience of patients. A significant portion of healthcare professionals and learners grapple with burnout, a condition characterized as "the state of mental and physical exhaustion caused by one's profession."[8] The literature indicates that burnout is quite common among physicians and healthcare trainees, with more than half of all individuals affected.[9,10] Physician burnout leads to increased medical errors, poor collegial relationships, and clinicians leaving medical practice earlier, all of which can affect the safety and satisfaction of patients as well as the broader healthcare system.[11–13] Women and underrepresented groups in healthcare experience discrimination, harassment, and microaggressions throughout their careers that lead to serious negative effects, including burnout and suicidal thoughts.[14–16] Inequities and disparities in access to and outcomes of healthcare across different groups of individuals exist.[17] And all of these challenges have been magnified by the SARS-CoV-2 coronavirus and the resultant COVID-19 global pandemic, which has led to immense upheaval and changes in the way healthcare is delivered and received.

As teachers, attending physicians must be exemplars of 21st-century hospital-based medicine for their learners and role models for the delivery of team-based and patient-centered care. This is no small feat, given the changes in recent years that have drastically complicated the task of serving as an attending physician.

What This Book Offers

Despite the obstacles facing physicians and trainees today, steadfast teaching attending physicians continue to inspire generation after generation of medical learners to both learn medicine and practice with compassion. These exemplary individuals, like the one mentioned in the beginning paragraphs of this chapter, serve as role models and show others the joy of medicine. We believe it is a worthwhile endeavor to understand the methods used by these outstanding individuals so that others may incorporate them into their own practices.

Over the years, the vital importance of clinical education has inspired dozens of studies aimed at measuring the effectiveness of various teaching programs and offering recommendations for how best to do the job. Most of the studies provide lists of personal attributes and approaches to teaching that are favored by current learners based on their answers to questionnaires. Often, these inquiries fail to consider the individual learner's level of education. Medical students, for example, tend to place a high value on attending kindness, whereas residents want attendings who will give them maximal autonomy.[18,19] In other inquiries, the work of attendings is observed and analyzed by other physicians. But both methods of study rely on just a single perspective, and neither looks at teaching as a practice that includes other healthcare team members or patients in the learning process. Many prior articles in the field of effective teaching have been written by white men, and their experience may not capture the approaches and techniques of attendings who identify as women or underrepresented minorities.

Our study used a different tactic. The attending referred to at the start of this chapter is one of 18 exemplary physician teachers from around the country whom the authors directly observed making rounds on their hospitals' wards. The 18 were also interviewed, as were their current team members (medical students, interns, and residents) and practicing physicians who had once been team members of the 18. By means of this in-depth, exploratory, qualitative approach integrating multiple perspectives, we have been able to describe how these great attendings go about creating an inspiring, effective learning environment tailored to the vastly altered requirements of the 21st-century hospital.

What makes this book particularly valuable for attending physicians (and those who one day will be) is that it goes beyond the listing of desirable teaching attributes that most previous studies have offered. It provides a close-up, detailed description of the specific strategies, methods, attitudes, and even language that the 18 outstanding physicians use in their interactions with learners and patients on the wards.

In the past decade, there have been relatively few publications—books or journal articles—that examine the new circumstances of attending physicians and their efforts to adapt to an ever-changing world. This book was created to begin to fill that vacuum to help new and seasoned attendings meet current challenges, take excellent care of hospitalized patients, and inspire generations of medical learners. In it, we ask three pivotal questions: What kind of learning environments do great attendings create? How do they foster these environments? And, how do they teach to and role model for learners at multiple levels to provide exceptional inpatient care?

Our Philosophy and Approach

To find the answers, we began with the assumption that teaching of any kind is a social process in which students are active participants, not simply passive recipients of knowledge. Through that ongoing interaction, attendings and their team members create a community of ideas, values, and meaning that eventually yields an in-depth understanding of their shared world.[20] Attending physicians role model effective interactions and navigation of social situations, seek to coach others rather than assert their authority, and work to mentor future physicians. To discover how this process functions at the highest level, we began by seeking out great attending physicians—specifically, those who rounded on general medicine wards regardless of their medical specialty. If we could really capture their educational methods, we believed that we could provide a uniquely helpful guide for other attendings.

Since there is no national ranking of attending physicians, we identified physicians for our study by asking for nominations from two groups: the chiefs of medicine or other high-level officials at some of the nation's leading medical schools, and individual experts who had won teaching awards or were medical education specialists. Medical schools, excellence aside, vary in their resources and in the backgrounds of their students, and we made sure our school selections reflected those facts.

In total, we obtained 102 nominees across two separate studies. Thereafter, we narrowed the lists, seeking to make sure that a diversity of geography, patient population, attending background (i.e., gender, race, ethnicity), and attending experience would be represented in the final groupings. That left 23 total possible participants, and 18 of them agreed to take part in our studies—not a small commitment on their part.[21,22]

We asked attendings to allow us to observe and take notes as they made ward rounds with their teams (see Figure 1.1). They were asked to sit down for individual interviews with us and to help us arrange further interviews with their current—and some of their former—learners. We, in turn, agreed that our observations and the participants' comments included in this book would not be identified with any individual person.

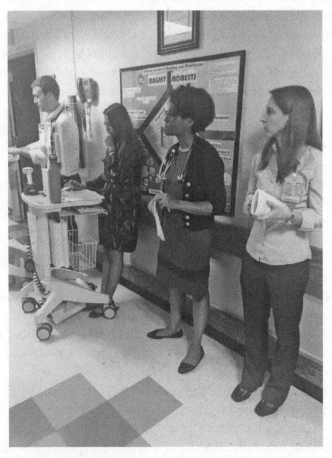

Figure 1.1 Attending physician listening intently during team rounds.

We should note that the 18 attendings were uncomfortable with the notion of themselves as "great" and only agreed to be part of our study because of its potential contribution to the field. During our interviews with them, they all suggested other physicians that we should be including. Indeed, we were and remain very conscious of the fact that our list of exemplary attendings leaves out a great many outstanding attendings across the country.

Social processes are hard to pin down, and the work of the attending physician is no exception. To understand the behavior and culture of these clinical teams, we spent time with their members in the context of their daily lives by going on rounds with them. In addition, our interviews provided multiple perspectives on the 18 attendings' modus operandi. Through interviews, the attendings revealed the methods they deemed most important to use while teaching. Interviews with current learners provided evidence of how the attendings' methods were perceived by their most important audience. The comments of physicians who had been taught by the 18 attendings allowed us to form a holistic view of the long-term effects of the attendings' approaches. It should be noted that, in some cases, we edited the transcripts of interviews with attendings and learners for length and clarity.

In all our dealings within the hospital setting, we had a distinct advantage: we were familiar with the territory. Two of our team members are physicians who frequently attend on the wards and who have roles as service leaders, and another team member is a medical anthropologist who has conducted multiple studies in healthcare settings.

Fair warning: we have not included ambulatory care in our research. We believed that there was a particular need for in-depth research into inpatient medical instruction in the modern hospital setting and that our particular skills and backgrounds were more oriented in that direction. In addition, inpatient and ambulatory settings emphasize different aspects of patient care. Because of this, we think that teaching in the ambulatory realm deserves its own study. Likewise, we focused all our attention on the general medicine wards rather than intensive care or inpatient subspecialty care units.

We felt this provided the most breadth and diversity in teaching opportunities. After all, patients who are admitted to general medicine services can have any number of different conditions.

In this book, we have organized the attributes and methods of the 18 attendings into several categories, starting with a general description of them as a group. We then show how the attendings create a sense of team and a supportive learning environment, how they teach, how they connect with patients, how they work amid crises, and how they navigate difficult issues at individual, local, societal, and international levels. We also provide approaches, techniques, and resources (all with supporting anecdotes) from our own practices to add additional perspective. At the end of each chapter, we itemize its main points and provide suggestions for further reading on these topics. A final chapter summarizes our key findings.

During our research, we saw that some techniques and personal qualities of the 18 attendings were at work in more than one aspect of their calling. A sense of humor, for example, was invaluable with both learners and patients. But the ways in which the attendings exercised their sense of humor differed considerably— self-deprecating, for example, or telling jokes, or subtle humor. We highlight various aspects of teaching and patient care that many of the learners and attendings emphasized as being effective and necessary in today's healthcare environments.

We found that not all the behaviors and techniques presented in the book were exhibited by every one of the 18 attendings. Different attendings had different lived experiences, and they brought to each situation their unique backgrounds and expertise. We describe common or shared techniques used by exemplary attendings, but we also seek to amplify underrepresented voices in medicine. In the pages that follow, we illustrate with examples from our observations and interviews just how the attendings harness their unique attributes and skills in their craft. It is in those very details, we believe, that readers will find the special contribution of this book.

Finally, each chapter follows a similar structure. Each will begin with a quote that exemplifies a key idea that will be discussed within. Chapters will also end with three main points that the reader should take away from the text. Finally, for those interested in learning more, we suggest several references for further reading, along with annotations.

Main Points

1. Time constraints, complex patients, healthcare crises, nuanced social situations, and the involvement of multiple healthcare disciplines have necessitated changes in the ways attending physicians teach and care for patients in the hospital.
2. Unlike prior research, our project focused on the context in which learning happens and selected the team (and the attending physician as the lead of the team) as the focus of research.
3. We directly observed and interviewed 18 attendings and their medical teams in order to provide detailed descriptions of the specific strategies, methods, and even language that the attendings use to teach their learners about medicine and about the compassionate care of human beings.

Further Reading

Desai SV, Asch DA, Bellini LM, et al. Education outcomes in a duty-hour flexibility trial in internal medicine. N Engl J Med 2018;378:1494–508.

    Accreditation Council for Graduate Medical Education (ACGME) duty-hour regulations affect residents' learning, job performance, and well-being. Prior to this publication, some had concerns that the inflexibility of these regulations was having a negative impact on physician training. As a way to test that idea, this study randomized 63 internal medicine residencies to either standard ACGME duty-hour regulations or to new, flexible regulations that had no shift length restrictions or minimum times off between shifts. The results revealed a divergence in opinion between residents and program directors participating in the study. For residents, flexible policies led to less satisfaction with their education as compared to their control counterparts under standard ACGME duty-hour regulations. This was true even though there were no significant differences between the two types of programs based on mean percentages of time spent in patient care versus education. Conversely, program directors were more satisfied with the flexible programs compared to those in ACGME standard programs.

Lehmann LS, Sulmasy LS, Desai S, ACP Ethics, Professionalism and Human Rights Committee. Hidden curricula, ethics, and professionalism: Optimizing clinical learning environments in becoming and being a physician: A position paper of the American College of Physicians. Ann Intern Med 2018;168:506–8.

According to this paper, there are four types of curricula that make up the learning environments of trainee physicians: formal (e.g., course content, competencies), informal (e.g., learning during rounds), hidden (not explicitly intended lessons; e.g., role modeling, respect for patients and colleagues), and null (what is not taught; e.g., social justice, patient advocacy). The American College of Physicians (ACP) here sets out its recommendations for best practices in teaching the hidden curriculum. These practices can be broken down into three recommendations. First, the informal and hidden curricula may not be consistent with the formal curricula, so they must be brought into line to take into account what is taught in the classroom so it can be reinforced—rather than undermined—at the bedside. Next, environment and culture should encourage "respect, inquiry, and honesty" while giving everyone in the program the tools and protections necessary to "raise concerns about ethics, professionalism, and care delivery." As with the first point, it is necessary to both teach and model patterns of behavior. Finally, the ACP recommends that leadership at these programs "create and sustain a strong ethical culture" that includes open discussion of ethical issues, explicitly leveraging values as part of decision-making, and placing the patient's well-being at the center of the professionalism taught to residents. In sum, the ACP recommends that the hidden curriculum be made visible and explicitly integrated into the curriculum of residency training programs.

Nickel WK, Weinberger SE, Guze PA, et al. Principles for patient and family partnership in care: An American College of Physicians position paper. Ann Intern Med 2018;169:796–9.

How we engage our patients and their families in the care model has long been a topic for debate and investigation. The ACP defines in this position paper its stance on three principles for partnering with patients and their families in patient care. First, patients and families should be treated with dignity and respect, which begins with recognizing them as individuals first, whose needs and concerns should be met with care and empathy. Next, the patient and their family should be actively engaged (to the level of their choosing) in all aspects of care planning and execution. In particular, care should not be done "to" or "for" a patient but "with" them, emphasizing the partnership between patient and provider. Finally, in order to improve our systems in the future, patients and families should collaborate with healthcare systems to improve them because the perspectives that patients and families provide may not be considered by healthcare providers. Patients and their families have increased the size of their roles in healthcare over the years, and that will only become more important as we further improve healthcare delivery.

Wachter RM, Verghese A. The attending physician on the wards: Finding a new homeostasis. JAMA 2012;308:977–8.

In this viewpoint, the authors, national leaders in academic medicine, present a picture of how the role and responsibilities of the attending have changed over time. They compare the teaching approach of older versus younger attendings and make the point that systems changes are necessary to accommodate these new approaches and requirements. For example, they emphasize that institutions should provide the support necessary to ensure a balance between teaching and providing patient care.

2

Unique Individuals, Shared Qualities

To find joy in work is to discover the fountain of youth.
—Pearl S. Buck

On one level, the nine men and nine women we observed and interviewed are a mixed bag. Some entered their training knowing they wanted to specialize in internal medicine, while others fell in love with a specialty during their training. One of the attendings began their career in psychiatry and another in orthopedic surgery. One was inducted into his state's football hall of fame, while another was a medical school valedictorian, and another served as a regular contributor to a variety of local and national media outlets.

The 18 each have unique styles of doctoring and teaching that frequently match with their personalities. One is a walking sunbeam, greeting passersby in the hallways and constantly joking with his team. Another conveys her warmth and humor in a quieter but no less effective manner. One is a self-described introvert but purposefully sets this characteristic aside with her team and her patients. During hospital rounds, some attendings are more hands-on with patients than others; some spend more time and energy on table rounds than do their counterparts. As one attending aptly stated: "if medicine is what you love doing, then find a style that works for you, even if it's different. . . . Embrace being different."

Teaching Inpatient Medicine. Second Edition. Nathan Houchens, Molly Harrod, and Sanjay Saint,
Oxford University Press. © Nathan Houchens, Molly Harrod, and Sanjay Saint 2023.
DOI: 10.1093/oso/9780197639023.003.0002

The Rise of Hospital Medicine

Yet, for all such differences, the 18 share some attributes. Most of them, for example, are hospitalists, members of history's fastest growing medical specialty. Hospitals in Great Britain and elsewhere had employed inpatient physicians for years, but they were rare in the United States. In 1996, an article in the *New England Journal of Medicine*, authored by Drs. Robert Wachter and Lee Goldman from the University of California at San Francisco, coined the term "hospitalist" and called for a new and more efficient division of labor— hospitalists for inpatients, primary care physicians for outpatients.[1] That arrangement, the authors argued, would assure that there would always be doctors on hand to care for hospital patients in need while freeing up primary care doctors to spend more time with their outpatients.

The seed was planted. From that standing start more than two decades ago, the ranks of hospitalists have swelled to more than 60,000.[2] They can be found in 75% of US hospitals and are not exclusively internists.[3] Today, there are orthopedic hospitalists, neurologic hospitalists, and obstetrics-gynecologic hospitalists, to name a few. Hospitalists can be found as CEOs of health systems, chief experience officers, information technology specialists, leaders of patient safety innovations, and directors of residency and medical school programs. The hospitalist movement has been a key element in the transformation of American hospitals and the teaching that takes place within them, aiding in the effort to shorten patients' stays, improve health and safety outcomes, and reduce costs. At the same time, hospitalists have played a crucial supporting role in the hospital industry's drive, under pressure from Washington, DC and the US public, toward higher quality, patient-centered care.[4]

Shared Qualities

The 18 attendings we studied share many other attributes. For example, they are very much alike in their full-hearted enthusiasm for the work. They are constantly striving to improve both their knowledge base and their teaching skills. And they have no hesitation admitting when they are wrong or simply don't know the answer to a question from a learner or patient.

This description of an attending by one of his former learners sums up the whole group: "No matter how many awards he might have won or how many other leadership positions he might have, ultimately, he was a doctor that loved taking care of patients and loved teaching—never there to sort of just get through something so that he could get on to something else, but very present and very excited about what he was doing."

Another of the 18 said of his calling, "I take great joy." He described the surprised reaction of hospital staffers when he showed up for work on holidays: "What are you doing here? It's Christmas." The attending's response: "I'm blessed. That's why I'm here."

Nothing is so powerful in accomplishing a challenging mission as a joyous commitment. As Steve Jobs put it, "The only way to do great work is to love what you do." The 18 attendings' enjoyment of teaching stems, in part, from their interest in other people— particularly young people who are treading the same path the attendings chose for themselves. They take pleasure in getting to know their team members, not just as the latest group of learners but as individuals, and conversations often extend beyond the hospital walls. In many cases, the attendings take on mentorship or coach roles with their learners, helping them to navigate their professional journeys.

One attending began rounds with inquiries to each team member of how they were feeling that day by asking, "Where are you on a scale of 1 to 5?" For each learner, the attending would ask follow-up questions: "What makes you feel like a 4.5 today? What makes you lose that other 0.5? What did you learn about in didactics yesterday afternoon?" When an embarrassed learner mentioned he had overslept that morning, the attending replied, "Your body must have really needed that." And, after each learner had shared, the attending shared her own score and reasons why. She was "solidly a 4.8" because she was working on getting 7 hours of sleep per night and had talked with her son about growth mindsets and imposter syndrome the previous evening, both activities she found personally meaningful. Later, upon hearing that social work had arranged for a patient to receive much-needed equipment in order to return home after discharge, the attending exclaimed, "*Now* I'm a 5-plus!"

All 18 attendings are highly intelligent, skilled, and knowledgeable physicians. "He just kind of knows a ton of [physical exam] maneuvers," a former learner said of his one-time attending, "some I have never even heard of. He just knows all of the data behind . . . the likelihood ratios for different things."

During the time they spend with their learners, the 18 are constantly looking for ways to share their knowledge (see Figure 2.1). We observed attendings who simply never stopped teaching their teams—before rounds began, with patients, walking from

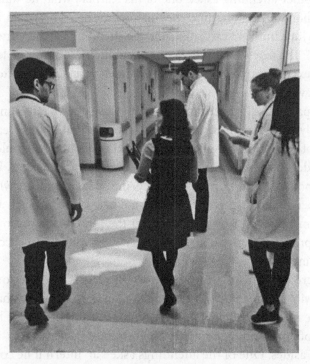

Figure 2.1 Attending physician utilizing every moment to teach.

patient to patient (including a mini-lecture in a stairwell), and after rounds. They possessed information that could repair bodies and save lives, and they were determined to share as much of it as possible.

Like anyone who loves their job, the 18 attendings are constantly alert for opportunities to do it better. They stay abreast of the medical literature and ferret out new facts wherever they are to be found. A former learner described his attending as "very curious," adding that he was "very much there to learn, to discover new things along with you." We heard one of the attendings telling his team that he had "checked the living daylights out of the literature" to follow up on a patient seen earlier. He finally decided to use a resource available to everyone: "I emailed the person that did the study and asked him about this." The upshot: "He said he's never seen this before."

Another attending asked one of his learners what he wanted to talk about. "I'm going into rheumatology," the learner told us, "so I did a little thing on vasculitis. And the attending sits there and takes notes." The teacher had no hesitation about becoming the learner. The next time anyone wants to know about vasculitis, the attending will have the answers.

As part of their determination to improve, the 18 attendings frequently gauged their own progress as well as that of their learners. One of them said he was "always thinking about what could have been done differently" after rounds were over. In this case, he was disappointed with himself for not being specific enough when he assigned some research. Self-assessment is a proven path to improvement. A 2015 study found that the more often you monitor your progress toward a goal, the more likely you are to succeed in attaining it.[5]

There are other attributes the 18 physicians have in common that will become apparent over the course of the next chapters. Of the attributes they had in common, it was their use of humor that often stood out. Often, their humor finds expression in quick asides. One of the attendings asked an intern if he could be more specific about the pathophysiology of a patient's problem.

When the intern passed, the attending turned the question to the other members of the team: "Who's feeling more specific?" Self-deprecating humor is also popular. An attending urged her team to, "Talk to me like I know nothing." After a pause, she continued, "Thank you for not saying that's how you always talk to me." Yet another mentioned that she appreciated the assistance of the hospital's interpreter services because, as she stated, "y'all *don't* want to see my Spanish."

For some, self-deprecating humor worked well to make the learning environment relaxed and comfortable; however, for others, it was a technique best avoided altogether. In particular, junior faculty—those individuals who had only recently become faculty attending physicians—who identified as female or as an underrepresented minority in medicine shared with us that learners, patients, and other healthcare team members would question their decisions as team leaders or lose trust in them if they used this type of humor. On the contrary, these individuals felt they needed to actively showcase their knowledge and abilities to be taken seriously, a concept we will return to shortly.

In the chapters ahead, we describe the perspectives of some underrepresented voices in healthcare and how they serve as teaching attendings. We explore the team environment and the approach to teaching favored by the 18 attending physicians, and we show the various methods they use to create and maintain that environment for each successive group of learners.

Main Points

1. Most of the attendings in this study were hospitalists, specializing in the care of patients within the hospital.
2. Although each attending had their own individual style of doctoring and teaching, we were able to identify qualities and attributes they all shared.
3. One of the most important attributes all the attendings shared was the conviction that they should never stop learning.

Further Reading

Omid A, Haghani F, Adibi P. Clinical teaching with emotional intelligence: A teaching toolbox. J Res Med Sci 2016;21:27.

Emotional intelligence—the degree to which we can process the emotional states of ourselves and others—is a required component of the teaching arts. Being able to adapt and appropriately respond to the emotional states of students or trainees is critical to success when engaged in learning activities. Based on the emotional intelligence concepts developed by Daniel Goleman, the authors identified 12 methods used by highly successful clinical teachers who were high in emotional intelligence. Built around the clinical teaching environment, the methods identified are as follows. Before rounds: know and manage your own emotional state; identify the survival needs of your patients, your team, and yourself; and create a motivational environment for all. During rounds: focus on developing and maintaining rapport; be transparent about your process as you teach through role modeling; teach in creative and emotionally engaging ways; leverage social and emotional learning; manage the social environment around your students and trainees to help them navigate; and ensure you foster a supportive environment for all. Then, after rounds, be sure to give interactive feedback while also evaluating your own teaching. Finally, be available to your learners and patients.

Salim SA, Elmaraezy A, Pamarthy A, Thongprayoon C, Cheungpasitporn W, Palabindala V. Impact of hospitalists on the efficiency of inpatient care and patient satisfaction: A systematic review and meta-analysis. J Community Hosp Intern Med Perspect 2019;9:121–34.

In the realm of medical specialties, the hospitalist is still a relative newcomer. Many researchers have studied the impact of a hospitalist-run care service by examining common quality measures (i.e., hospital length of stay, cost, readmission rate, mortality, and patient satisfaction) and comparing those to non–hospitalist-run care services. The systematic review and meta-analysis conducted by Salim and colleagues indicates a significant reduction in length of stay for hospitalist services. Other measures for hospitalist-run services were comparable to or slightly better than non–hospitalist-run services, indicating that hospitalist-run services are more efficient compared to non–hospitalist-run services (in terms of length of stay and patient satisfaction) while providing comparable care quality.

Wachter RM, Goldman L. The emerging role of "hospitalists" in the American health care system. N Engl J Med 1996;335:514–7.

In this sounding board, the emerging role and potential future of the hospitalist in the American healthcare system is discussed. The authors describe the varying reasons why they believe the hospitalist specialty will flourish. These reasons include cost pressures, the need for physicians who can provide care for a large panel of patients, and the ability of hospitalists to utilize immediately available resources to quickly respond to changes in a patient's condition. Wachter and Goldman also outline several objections facing the hospitalist model.

3
Underrepresented Voices

Our ability to reach unity in diversity will be the beauty and the test of our civilization.

—Mahatma Gandhi

Individuals from historically marginalized or minoritized groups have long faced many challenges. In medicine, women and underrepresented minorities (defined by the Association of American Medical Colleges as "those racial and ethnic populations that are underrepresented in the medical profession relative to their numbers in the general population"[1]) especially face difficulties like discrimination, unconscious bias, and harassment from patients, family members, supervisors, colleagues, and other healthcare employees.[2–5] Inappropriate behaviors and biases may arise because of a person's visible and less visible identities and may be based in age, gender identity, race, color within race, religion, perceived ability, and many other features and characteristics.

Among many examples, women and underrepresented minorities are often mistakenly identified as non-physician care team members or assumed to hold non-leadership positions. Meanwhile, individuals who identify or are frequently coded as both men and Caucasian—a sociodemographic group that has historically predominated Western medicine—are often assumed to be physician leaders, regardless of training level or their role on the team. And historically, this assumption was unsurprising because the number of women matriculating into medical school in the 1960s

Teaching Inpatient Medicine. Second Edition. Nathan Houchens, Molly Harrod, and Sanjay Saint, Oxford University Press. © Nathan Houchens, Molly Harrod, and Sanjay Saint 2023. DOI: 10.1093/oso/9780197639023.003.0003

was only 6%.[6,7] However, this number rose to 55% by 2021,[8] and yet women still make up only 41% of associate professors and 27% of full professors (based on data from the Association of American Medical Colleges).[9]

Knowing that these challenges exist, we sought to better understand and document the strategies used by outstanding female and underrepresented teaching attending physicians to navigate gender- and race/color-based challenges. While there is ample literature discussing the types of challenges faced by women and underrepresented minorities—even including how institutions can work to resolve these challenges—little has been studied on the personal techniques used to combat such issues. Since the first edition of this book, our team followed six additional exemplary attendings who identified as women (some of whom also identified as minorities underrepresented in medicine), conducting observations during teaching rounds and following up with interviews and focus groups with former learners taught under these attendings.[7]

Our purpose in this chapter is not to dissect every discrete challenge faced (it would be impossible to capture every individual's unique lived experience) nor give a universal formula for "solving" them (because one does not exist). Rather, we provide an overview of strategies that exemplary women and underrepresented minority leaders have employed to mitigate these challenges. We do this by placing a focus on the women and underrepresented minorities from whom we have learned. Until the day that these struggles have dissipated, our hope is that their strategies may be known, built upon, and taught to empower those who face these challenges more often than perhaps we are aware.

Mitigating Bias and Harassment

Through directly observing attending interactions with both learners and patients during rounds, as well as interviews with the attendings themselves and their current and former learners, we identified overlapping strategies that female and underrepresented minority attendings employ in their interactions. While the techniques they use to address their respective and, at times, intersecting challenges may overlap, we will discuss female attendings and underrepresented attendings separately. We begin with strategies used to specifically navigate gender-based challenges, categorized into three main themes.[7]

1. Female attendings actively position themselves as physician team leaders.
2. Female attendings consciously work to manage gender-based stereotypes.
3. Female attendings intentionally identify and embrace their unique qualities.

Active Positioning as Team Leader

If you speak with a female physician, it is likely she can tell you about a time when she was mistaken for or assumed to be a nurse, physical therapist, technician, or any member of the care team other than the physician. Or perhaps she may recall the time she was asked to do tasks that are misaligned with her duties as a physician. This has led to women feeling invisible in professional settings like healthcare. One attending specifically called this out: "I think every woman in this role has been mistaken for a different caretaker role, so lots of requests for nursing help. I'm sure I have taken more patients off of bed pans and brought more cups of water than maybe some of my male counterparts." Learners made note of the phenomenon as well. One former learner commented, "I think that, like many times on our team, you know, she is a Black female and they [patients] would look to the White male med student as the attending when we would walk in the room. And so, that's awkward."

Facing this common occurrence, several female attendings choose to wear white coats on rounds and during each patient encounter, visually marking themselves as the attending and one of the physicians

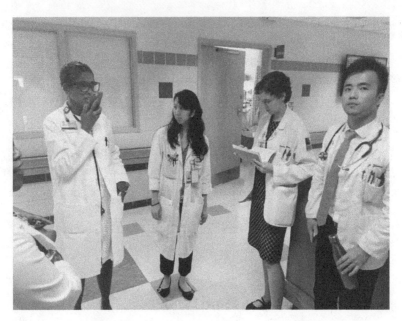

Figure 3.1 Female attending and team members wearing white coats.

on the team (see Figure 3.1). On one observation of rounds at the hospital, we found that all of the women and none of the men on one particular team wore white coats while seeing patients together. A former learner commented on this strategy: "I have noticed—and someone actually told me—that, like, female attendings will make more of a point to wear their white coat all the time and that is because they walk into rooms and then, [are misidentified] as a nurse or called 'honey' or things like that."

Not everyone buys into the concept that white coats clearly distinguish women as leaders of teams. Some feel that the gender stereotypes run deep and strong and are not alleviated by simple visual cues. One former learner who identified as female reflected, "I don't think it [wearing a white coat] helps. I have gotten—even if you introduce yourself as a doctor, I have patients who still think I'm a nurse a lot of the times, and then they think sometimes even if they have a male nurse, they think that person may be a doctor, so I think it's like the societal conception."

We also found that patients and their family members expected men to be team leaders, and, therefore, attendings would respond by clearly introducing all team members by both name and role, including themselves. As patients assumed or confused roles, attendings would gently redirect and remind them. This bias was not specific to the patient population. Decision-making was more often questioned by other healthcare employees when the attending was a woman. One attending described how she is sometimes talked to by consultant colleagues—"Who is your attending? Let me talk with them"—assuming that the female attending was not truly the person in charge.

Power struggles like these were also felt with nurses, learners, and others. One learner described a scenario in which conflict existed between a nurse and female attending, explaining that the attending was treated by the nurse "differently . . . questioning [the] decisions." In this case, an extra dose of confidence was utilized at the bedside by the attending. Asserting ideas and medical decisions, and being more direct than their male counterparts, were strategies often used in overcoming these challenges. Yet sometimes this assertiveness was received negatively, as we will discuss in a moment.

Questioning and second-guessing of decisions led several female attendings to experience self-doubt, dubbed by many as *imposter syndrome*. Gender dynamics played a significant role in this challenge, although gender was not the only identity that contributed to imposter syndrome. More on that in a minute.

Conscious Work to Manage Gender-Based Stereotypes

During our interviews, when we discussed how female attendings navigate interactions at work, it became clear that this "extra dose of confidence" is a fine line to walk. Gender-based challenges, ranging from microaggressions to discrimination to overt sexual harassment, were often described, and attendings explained feeling that they were walking a very thin tightrope between being perceived as "too nice" and "too aggressive." These stereotypical qualities—with kindness and compassion considered feminine, and aggression and confidence considered masculine—have been well described.[10] Extremes in either direction carried negative connotations. Likewise, the perception and interpretation of these qualities also depends on gender. For instance, men may be allowed to be more aggressive, which is often interpreted as being "confident," whereas if women are perceived to be aggressive—even mildly so—it may be interpreted as being "angry." During one attending interview, we heard the following powerful comments:

> I think for women attendings, if you are very competent and you just do your job in kind of a nondescript way, you will be deemed "nice," and it's usually the first adjective that women get. And I give feedback to women on my teams all the time that you want to be nice, but you don't want that to be the first thing somebody says about you.

This tightrope act seemed toughest to hold when inappropriate and harmful comments were made, such as "You're too young to be a physician," or "You're too pretty." Though perhaps not intended as an insult or slight, comments such as these have important and problematic effects for individuals at all stages of their professional careers in medicine. For instance, among all levels of medical trainees, 59% experienced some form of harassment or discrimination,[11] and, among first year medical students, 77% reported microaggressions.[12] A study of surgical resident physicians noted that patients and families are the most common source of inappropriate behaviors and uncovered the staggering statistic that those who report inappropriate behaviors a few times per month were three times more likely to experience professional burnout and even suicidal thoughts.[13] Yet the effects don't stop there. Nearly two-thirds of female faculty physicians and nearly half of male faculty reported sexual harassment from patients and patients' families.[14] These unwanted and unwarranted behaviors are pervasive, and their effects are profound.

Actions taken by female teaching attendings to mitigate harassing and microaggression scenarios included attendings distancing themselves from their feminine characteristics and redirecting attention away from their personal and physical characteristics and toward their professional qualities. Intentional planning of how to carry oneself was at the forefront of the mind for these attendings. One voiced, "[I] purposefully [avoid] doing things that are kind of classically female in order to make sure that people respect and respond to me as a physician, rather than as a female physician."

Additionally, these attendings also considered how much makeup or jewelry to wear, knowing that these decisions might impact the way they would be treated. According to some of our attendings, more attention to makeup or jewelry typically resulted in being taken less seriously as a physician. Similarly, select types of attire could spark inappropriate and unwanted comments from others. "I know that doesn't happen with my male colleagues," one physician remarked. As a result, female attendings were careful in selecting their outward ensemble, from clothing to personal appearance and even facial expressions, to minimize their femininity.

Identifying and Embracing Unique Qualities

The difficult thing for women is that you have to figure out— "How can I be myself?" . . . And I think that is, "What is your Whitney Houston? What is your jam? What should you be doing that nobody else can do like you?" Figure it out because, once you do, it's going to open you all the way up. You are going to become more confident in everything you do, and the team is going to see you differently.

We heard this from one attending who spoke of embracing one's unique qualities, leaning in to what makes you, you. While embracing the true authentic self is good advice for individuals of any gender, it may be more necessary for female attendings, who may feel they cannot conform to typical masculine expectations in medicine. Areas of expertise, communication style, teaching methods, to name a few, are all domains that these female attendings had dug deep to identify and embrace. These qualities, it seemed, were often what led learners to remember these notable attendings even after years had passed.

As briefly mentioned before, even with mitigation strategies, challenges faced by women are bound to lead to questions of adequacy and worth. Fearful feelings of being "found out" or exposed as a fraud often keep individuals from truly embracing their unique qualities. Frequent questioning from peers, concern over perception based on appearance, and toeing the line of effective confidence undoubtedly add up and contribute to internalized imposter syndrome. One attending remarked, "And I still take things personally. You can even get 20 good evals and one bad eval and then you are like, clearly, this is—the bad one is the accurate one, and I am this!"

Yet this same attending recalled, after winning their fourth straight teaching award, "It was just like something changed in me. . . . Maybe you *are* a good attending. Maybe you are doing something that is resonating with a unique class of medical students year after year." Of course, not all will have the reassurance and validation of award recognition (especially since biases may be present in award selection processes), but it goes to show that even the most advanced physician in their field may experience feelings of doubt. Pushing back on these thoughts and feelings entailed acknowledgment of imposter syndrome and, for some, repeating positive, self-affirming messages—something that everyone can do. More than one attending noted that choosing to "release" doubts was personally and professionally effective. "It's being able to brush that stuff off," advised one attending. "You know, let it go and not dwelling too much on it."

When individual efforts and self-affirmations don't seem to be enough to lessen the imposter syndrome, there may be a role for female mentors and sponsors, a subject we return to in Chapter 9. Some of our great attendings noted that a support network of women—intentional in promoting one another, their achievements, and their work—improves not only imposter syndrome feelings but also advances an individual's career by distributing and publicizing their successes. Indeed, a whole other book could be written on the importance of mentorship—and has.[15]

Similar Challenges, Unique Experiences

The same issues that arise as a result of gender bias often manifest similarly because of a person's race, color within race, and ethnicity. At times, these can be difficult to distinguish from those faced by women, and yet, each individual's lived experience is unique and cannot be generalized.

Some attending physicians who identified as underrepresented minorities told us that they grapple with the ways in which they are (or are not) recognized and promoted as leaders in their institutions. One attending, commenting on the types of roles that are offered, mentioned, "Maybe there's promotion [recognition and career advancement] in so far as 'do you want to be on the committee to attract more underrepresented minorities to medicine?' Sure. There's those offers but, you know, like do you want to run the fellowship? That's, I think, a lot harder to climb . . . as a minority but also as a female."

Teasing out the root causes for imposter syndrome proved to be especially difficult for some attendings who had the intersecting identities of being a woman and an underrepresented minority.

> Because I feel like in the back of my mind—it still comes that I know it's irrational a little bit—but part of me is like, am I getting all these opportunities because I'm female, because I'm a minority? I know that I am a good physician. I know I can teach. I get that. . . . I have been given lots of great opportunities, and part of me wants to make sure that I'm truly deserving of it.

Our teaching attendings shared with us their disappointment that these strategies were even necessary: that racism, sexism, ableism, ageism, and discrimination based on visible and not-so-visible identities persist. Yet, in the same breath, they also shared how it had become so commonplace that it was almost stitched into the fabric of their lives; they had "learned to live with it" as a coping mechanism.

How, then, did our attendings confront these pervasive biases and prejudices for their teams? It tended to start from within, using their own purposeful responses to inappropriate or problematic comments. The Greek philosopher Epictetus said, "We cannot choose our external circumstances, but we can always choose how we respond to them."[16] Our attendings embraced this concept fully. "I think nobody can make you feel inferior without your consent," one said with a smile. "It's like what Eleanor Roosevelt said. I've had that conversation with many, many women who look like me in this setting."

The attendings we interviewed each took their role model status seriously when it came to advocating for their learners—particularly those who were of marginalized and minoritized groups—and showing patients new ways of thinking. When talking about patient-initiated inappropriate comments, one attending reflected, "I don't think most of the time that it's intentional or mean-hearted; it's just ignorance and what they are used to. I'm just trying to show them otherwise." Another attending who identified as Asian and who worked in a rural community commented, "I don't look like somebody who can talk John Deere tractors, but I try to, you know, connect in whatever way and role model that for my team, too."

For some who identified as women or underrepresented minorities, conversations with learners entailed explicit discussion on how to respond (rather than react) to instances of discriminatory behavior from anyone.

So, when I sat down with that resident that was on our team today who looks like me and I said, "Look: there are going to be people who meet you and when they meet you, when they see you, they are going to have an idea in their head—not even because they are being mean, but because of their own unconscious bias—of just how good you can be. Just how good. You can only be so good. You can't be quite as good as this next person. And so . . . you have an opportunity to maybe teach them something new."

Audre Lourde, an American writer, feminist, and civil rights activist said, "It is not our differences that divide us. It is our inability to recognize, accept, and celebrate those differences."[17] As with female attendings, those who identified as underrepresented minorities in medicine advised future generations of physicians to embrace their differences, to lift them up rather than to assimilate to traditional expectations. This may apply to how one communicates with others, as evidenced by this passage from one of the attendings we interviewed.

> I think I have a different . . . communication style maybe? Maybe less formal, and I have had comments from colleagues and prior learners that my style in the room is different as well. It's respectful but not . . . I don't sort of dictate things to patients. Again, it's a conversation, so, I realized that about myself very early, and when I was in training, [you] had to conform to whatever environment you were in. But when I got out into practice and realized that I could be myself and people were responsive to that, then that just perpetuated my current style. . . . And I like to be different.

As we continue to discuss the effects exemplary teaching attendings have on learners, it is worth noting that attendings recognized that how they perceive themselves—and their authenticity—impacts the experiences of their team members. One attending summed it up this way:

> I can speak for African American experiences because that's my background—that I have spent a lot of years just trying to assimilate and just trying to, you know, stay as neutral as possible. . . . And I did that when I was an intern for about 6 months, and it was absolutely exhausting! And then, finally, I was just like, you know what? My high school was 95% Black, 5% Mexican, zero percent anything else. I went to a historically Black college. Then I went to a historically Black medical school. I really don't know how to assimilate, and it will exhaust me to

do so. And so, for me, I think it's great for my residents because I'm really comfortable in my skin.

The Whole Picture

Many healthcare systems recognize the need to improve institutional culture in order to better the experiences of women and underrepresented minorities in medicine. Many times, this has been done through establishing sexual harassment policies, striving to ensure diversified recruitment, retaining underrepresented faculty and staff, and working to better integrate the many domains of life and work. Our findings support the need for systemic change but also dive deeper to identify the strategies that female and underrepresented minority attendings use to navigate biases and stereotype-based challenges. We acknowledge that these strategies may not be taken up by, or even appeal to, every individual. As our attendings have highlighted, authenticity and being true to oneself are critical.

A somewhat surprising result from this study was female attendings' emphasis on teaching their strategies to female learners and much less focus on their own personal responses. Often, when asked how one handles a particular gender-based issue, what we heard was how the attending instructs learners to handle the given scenario while minimizing it for themselves. This could be due to an inherent discomfort when speaking about moments of harassment or bias; however, the attendings reflected a genuine care for learners who would likely face these challenges. Far less tolerance was shown toward gender bias when it impacted learners than when it was directed toward the attendings or someone more "established" in their role. Most attendings voiced a strong desire to equip young physicians with the tools needed to combat these challenges, echoing their commitment to teaching.

Issues of harassment, bias, power struggles, and labeling have long existed in the workplace. Through actively positioning themselves as leaders, consciously working to manage stereotypes, and embracing their unique qualities, many of our attendings have defined their own approaches to navigating these challenges. Any person in the workplace around you may, at this very moment, be walking the tightrope of kindness and assertiveness so that their authority can be appropriately recognized and appreciated. Until the workplace culture shifts to one of true equity, we hope these strategies will help in both understanding and mitigating the challenges that so many face daily.

No one person can provide comprehensive and quality care alone. In the next chapter, we explore how medical teams arose through history. More importantly, we examine the ways in which exemplary teaching attendings build their teams: how they serve as coaches, build reciprocal trust, get to know their learners as people, and foster effective teamwork with all the myriad individuals who are taking care of the patient.

Main Points

1. In medicine, just as in other aspects of society, marginalized and minoritized groups face multiple challenges including discrimination, unconscious biases, and harassment. In particular, these challenges are felt disproportionately by women and underrepresented minorities.

2. Outstanding teaching attendings navigate stereotype-based biases by actively positioning themselves as leaders of physician teams, consciously working to manage stereotypes, and intentionally identifying and embracing their own unique qualities. It is particularly important to them to equip learners with these same skills.

3. Imposter syndrome occurs when an individual doubts their own abilities and maintains a persistent internalized fear of being exposed as fraudulent. Some attendings recognize this and consciously work to shed their doubts.

Further Reading

LaDonna KA, Ginsburg S, Watling C. "Rising to the level of your incompetence": What physicians' self-assessment of their performance reveals about the imposter syndrome in medicine. Acad Med 2018;93:763–8.

Imposter syndrome—feeling unqualified to hold the work position one does despite years of education and training—is a common experience among those who work in medicine. Errors during the provision of care can create anxiety and guilt—but especially self-doubt. This qualitative study examined the experiences of 28 physicians concerning their perspective on underperformance. Investigators found that physicians commonly experienced imposter syndrome. Interviewees who experienced this effect tended to be at the extreme end of the self-doubt scale, unable to receive positive feedback from colleagues to shore up their insecurities. This study reveals that all physicians can experience imposter syndrome, regardless of where they stand in their careers. Key contributors that can trigger this self-doubt are frequent transitions between roles or new professional challenges. These are, unfortunately, common occurrences within medicine. Recognizing struggling trainees or colleagues is critical to creating space to share and receive support for real or perceived underperformance.

Pololi LH, Civian JT, Brennan RT, Dottolo AL, Krupat E. Experiencing the culture of academic medicine: Gender matters, a national study. J Gen Intern Med 2013;28:201–7.

Though women have consistently made up 30–50% of medical school classes (at the time of this study), female representation in academic medicine remains very low. Women's careers advance substantially more slowly than those of men. This study aimed to identify key outcomes using factor analysis to generate culture dimensional scales. The authors then used the factor analysis to compare between genders. Compared to their male counterparts, female faculty indicated a lower sense of belonging and self-efficacy for advancing their careers. Women perceived that there was less gender equity and less organizational effort to address this inequality (e.g., via diversity, equity, and inclusion efforts). Finally, this study showed that female faculty perceived their institutions as less family-friendly and less aligned to their personal values. In all other factors, this study identified no differences between men and women (e.g., level of engagement and aspirations for leadership, amount of ethical or moral distress, perception of the institution's commitment to developing faculty and improve faculty support).

Shankar M, Albert T, Yee N, Overland M. Approaches for residents to address problematic patient behavior: Before, during, and after the clinical encounter. J Grad Med Educ 2019;11:371–4.

Problematic patient behavior, particularly in the form of microaggressions, have for too long been considered a "rite of passage" during medical training. Rather than address the issue—which contributes to patient avoidance behavior, worse work performance, and, ultimately, burnout—the training that exists to handle these situations is part of the "hidden curriculum." The authors of this perspective argue that the hidden curriculum in this instance must be formalized and brought into the explicit curriculum. This perspective offers concrete action steps to do so. First, attending physicians can create a safe space·in which their students can learn to address these situations. Attendings can elicit team input on how to respond to problematic behaviors, offering to step in or allowing the trainees to address the issue. Having a commitment from the entire team to support one another in these instances will provide a broader sense of safety for trainees. During the encounter, de-escalation techniques can help keep the patient encounter productive and professional. Finally, debriefing with the team can help work through any lingering negative emotions and help identify strategies for better future encounters. Team reflection on patient encounters may reduce the likelihood of burnout.

4

Building the Team

*The power of one, if fearless and focused, is formidable, but
the power of many working together is better.*

—Gloria Macapagal Arroyo

One of the outstanding 18 attending physicians shared with us the joy she brings to the hospital and to her learners each day. She also noted the considerable time and energy she devotes to ensure a cohesive team while teaching.

> I love what I do. I love being on the wards, and so I want to convey that to my team, and I want them to love it too, and the excitement of it. So, when I go to teach, first of all, I want to understand who my learners are. I want to know what their objectives are, what their goals are, so I can tailor [my teaching] to what they might be interested in. I definitely prefer a small group. I think that's why I like teaching on the clinical wards.

The attendings we observed told us—and showed us—how seriously they take their responsibility to establish and maintain close-knit teams, cooperative rather than competitive, with team members concerned for their patients and for each other. Such teams perform more effectively on the wards, and their members do a better job of learning to become outstanding doctors themselves. That double obligation to minister to the sick and to learn has a checkered history—as does the role of the attending physician within the medical team.

Teaching Inpatient Medicine. Second Edition. Nathan Houchens, Molly Harrod, and Sanjay Saint, Oxford University Press. © Nathan Houchens, Molly Harrod, and Sanjay Saint 2023.
DOI: 10.1093/oso/9780197639023.003.0004

A Brief History of Physician Teams in the United States

Back when the United States was born, doctors started their careers as apprentices, gradually learning their masters' techniques for pulling teeth and bleeding the sick. Toward the end of the 18th century, the University of Pennsylvania medical school began providing a year of hospital study and clinical practice after completion of apprenticeship; it was the nation's first internship. Some would-be doctors were also able to further their study in Europe, which was more sophisticated than the United States in terms of medical education.

The stage was set for the widespread development of university-sponsored, high-quality medical schools, with access to hospitals for clinical training on the charity wards. But, as apprenticeship waned over the next century, a host of for-profit, ersatz medical schools popped up, most providing the bare modicum of classwork and little or no clinical experience. Graduates gained that experience on the backs, as it were, of their initial, unlucky patients. With a hint of better days to come, the Johns Hopkins Hospital opened in 1889 and soon began offering the nation's first residency for pursuit of specialty training—an opportunity that was reserved, however, for only the very top students. Medical school alone was no longer viewed as sufficient preparation for practice.

As the country grew in the first years of the 20th century, rapidly expanding hospitals relied more and more on house officers: physicians in training who were both reliable and inexpensive. Their primary reimbursement was room and board within the hospital, which was how they came to be known as "residents." Over countless hours each day, they performed many of the hospital's menial tasks, but they were also able to learn. Time was set aside for interns and residents to examine patients and, especially at teaching hospitals, to treat them—all under the strict direction of the attending physician.

In 1914, the American Medical Association issued a list of 603 hospitals approved for the teaching of interns, and over the next few decades, graduate medical education flourished. "Most faculty took a keen interest in teaching, advising, and mentoring," Kenneth M. Ludmerer comments in his book, *Time to Heal*. "House officers could not help feeling close to—and supported by—their instructors."[1] Over weeks at a time, house officers were able to get to know and treat patients without such modern pressure points as length of stay metrics and reimbursement rules.

The Department of Veterans Affairs (VA) has played a key role in medical training. As one of us wrote several years ago to commemorate Veterans Day,

Two out of three medical doctors in practice in the US today received some part of their training at a VA hospital. The reason dates to the end of World War II. The VA faced a physician shortage, as almost 16 million Americans returned from war, many needing health care. At the same time, many doctors returned from World War II and needed to complete their residency training. The VA and the nation's medical schools thus became partners. In fact, the VA is the largest provider of health care training in the country, which increases the likelihood that trainees will consider working for the VA once they finish.[2]

After World War II, hospitals began a long period of exponential growth, spurred by government support and insurers' open-ended, fee-for-service payments. In the 1980s, however, Medicare and other insurers called a halt to these lucrative fee-for-service arrangements. Henceforth, hospitals would receive a fixed payment per patient depending on their diagnosis. The longer a patient remained in the hospital, the less likely the hospital would be to recoup its expenses. As a result, hospitals began shortening patients' stays which, at times, deleteriously affected house staff training. Learners had less time with any given patient and, when limits were placed on their daily duty hours in 2003, less time with patients overall.

Teaching hospitals became more corporate and competitive, more intent on market share and cost efficiency. The close, supportive connection between attendings and learners eroded as faculty applied for remunerative research grants, many times at the expense of their teaching. Critics charged that house staff were spending fewer hours on the wards and at the bedside in favor of the classroom and technological teaching aids. As a Boston University professor put it, "The wealth of bedside teaching opportunities is diminishing with rapid patient discharges, overabundance, and over-reliance on technology."[3]

The 18 outstanding attendings we followed know how to cope with the challenges of today's hospital. Their ability to build and maintain competent, cooperative teams is an essential part of that know-how.

The Attending Physician Serves as the Coach of the Team

Sadly, as Ken Bain[4] notes in his book, *What the Best College Teachers Do*, "teaching is one of those human endeavors that seldom benefits from its past. Great teachers emerge, they touch the lives of their students, and . . . subsequent generations must discover anew the wisdom of their practices" (p. 3). But discover they do, and Bain concludes on a similarly positive note, convinced that "good teaching can be learned" (p. 21). One of the current learners described his attending's approach.

> The most junior person has to be in charge. The medical student is the one who is going into the room and asking the questions and doing the history and the physical. And when the attending comes in the afternoon and he wants to run the list, that medical student is the person who does it. It's not, you know, a five-minute job with the senior. It's everybody . . . taking care of their patients; they are in charge.

At the core of their team-building skills is a firm determination to make it all about the team and to keep their own role to that of a watchful, benevolent coach. They have completely eschewed the physician-centric teams of the past. They see themselves as coaches more than bosses, fellow lifelong learners more than authorities, since they expect all members of the team to carry the torch for excellent patient care. Here's how one of the attendings gets that message across:

I really teach like I practice, which is in a team style, so that discussions are discussions and conversations around practice decisions. I think that's the approach I take, is a team effort. We teach each other and I'm there to guide and redirect as needed but not to dictate so much how we approach things, and I think that's reflected in my teaching style as well.

Our 18 attendings' approach to teaching is the very opposite of malicious "pimping," the posing of purposefully esoteric, unanswerable questions by an attending to demonstrate their superiority.[5] They want to encourage harmony within the group, not sow discord. In fact, when our 18 attendings ask questions of their teams, they are frequently directed first toward the team member with the least clinical experience. "He would ask us questions that it would be clear the [medical] students would be able to answer," a former learner recalled. "It bred this environment of inclusion." For these attendings, every member of a clinical team is equal in terms of opportunities to learn, to carry the torch, and to teach.

Team Structures Foster Learning and Patient Care

Learning is not limited solely to the learner who is presenting the patient on rounds. Team members benefit from discussions of the other members' patients, which include the right decisions, the mistakes, and all the gray areas in between. Attendings and patients benefit as well. "You are going to pick up on things for your patient that I won't pick up on," one attending tells his team. Another made the desire and need for team-based collaboration explicit: "I like it to be interactive. I don't like to be the sole talker. So, I want to have conversation and debate and information sharing; so, very much a group activity where everybody is involved in taking care of the patient and figuring out what we can best do for them."

Our 18 attendings want as many members of their team as possible to participate each day during rounds. For one, it allows attendings to evaluate how the various members are progressing in their medical decision-making and clinical work. For another, having the team participate together on rounds fosters cohesion. Members get to know each other better, share concerns and jokes, recognize strengths and weaknesses, and make space for both (see Figure 4.1). They help each other study, they have each other's backs when challenges arise, and they have fun. As legendary Michigan football coach Bo Shembechler emphasized: "The team, the team, the team."[6] A cohesive team, the attendings believe, does a better job of caring for patients.

One of the 18 described a most positive outcome from this approach: "There is this incredible efficiency when the whole team sees the patient together and figures out the plan, and there is no 'I will see him later in the day' or 'We'll close the loop later on and see what the attending thinks.' We are done by 10:30 with our decision-making."

The team structure as a model for organizing work has, in recent years, achieved broad acceptance in industry. Studies have demonstrated that teams performing high-intensity tasks make fewer mistakes than individual workers.[7] This finding aligns with modern

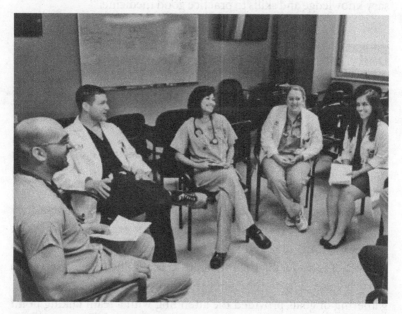

Figure 4.1 Members of a team getting to know each other before rounds.

educational theory, which tends to identify two basic varieties of learning. The first is knowledge acquisition, enabling the individual to reproduce the information studied. The second is knowledge gained through participation in a dynamic community of practice,[8] a team; the individual's professional identity is defined and refined throughout the learning process. Team learning has an obvious side benefit for hospitals, where collaboration among clinicians (during team-based resuscitation efforts for a patient suffering in-hospital cardiac arrest, for example) is so vital. And, as we noted earlier, clinical teams can bring more brainpower to bear on a patient's care than that provided by a single practitioner. In his book *The Diversity Bonus: How Great Teams Pay Off in the Knowledge Economy*, Scott E. Page[9] describes that identity-diverse teams—those groups of individuals who have diversity of race, ethnicity, gender, religion, and so on—contribute to enhanced team performance through cognitive diversity, provided that the work culture is inclusive. But the singular achievement of clinical team education, properly pursued, is the creation of principled, humane physicians who have absorbed the necessary knowledge and skills to practice good medicine.[10]

Daily Team-Building

Eliciting Goals and Setting Expectations on the First Day

Each in their own way, the attendings start team building on their first day. One attending has members write down three goals: (1) something they particularly want to learn about, (2) something they want to see fixed within the hospital, and (3) something personal they want to achieve. A former learner offered an example: "I will cook dinner five times during this rotation." The sharing of goals began the process of introducing the members to each other. It also served to alert the attending to the members' clinical interests. Not least, the gathering of goals provided the attending with a team talking point for the future, as in: "Hey, Jesse, how many of those dinners have you cooked so far?"

Each attending has their own priorities and preferences for team dynamics and daily activities. One attending, at the first session with her team, stated some of her priorities, including her preference for short presentations at the bedside in the interest of efficiency. Then she asked the senior residents how they wanted to run rounds (see Figure 4.2). What were some of the arrangements or formats they

---

Dr. O'Rorke's Wonderful World of Wards

No-blame culture

1. I expect mistakes to be made
2. I will always support you
   a. If you are honest
   b. You play as a team member
3. Ask questions if something is not clear

Pre-rounds

1. Interns and students will arrive early enough to:
   a. Collect all data
   b. See patient
   c. Obtain sign out from night float
   d. Formulate preliminary assessment and plan

Work Rounds with Resident

1. If time allows, resident should see all patients with intern and students
   a. Allows for modeling, teaching and direct feedback
2. Card flipping may be done if pt is stable with no active issues, but resident MUST see pt at some point before attending rounds.
3. Assessment and plan should be formulated
4. Start discharge process on pts that you feel are ready to leave
5. Order tests and call consults if you feel appropriate
6. End work rounds on time to allow attendance at morning report

Attending Rounds

1. Be prepared with assessment and plan for each patient
2. Discuss pts in the following order:
   a. Unstable
   b. Ready for discharge
   c. Need help with clinical decision
3. Rounds may vary based on census and acuity of pts
4. Dress neatly and professionally
5. Rounds will end on time. If necessary I will see remaining patients with the resident or on my own.

Figure 4.2 Handout of attending expectations of various team members' roles and responsibilities.

Progress Notes
BE VERY CAREFUL IF COPY and PASTING-make sure to update as needed

Roles
Attending
> Coach/counselor/teacher
> I am available 24/7
> Please notify me if:
>> A patient dies
>> A patient suddenly worsens
>> You decide a patient is ready for discharge
>> A patient wants to leave AMA
>> Conflicts with other services

Resident
> Responsible for all the patients
> Leader of the team
> Coordinator
> Expeditor
> Thinker, researcher, reader
> Provides education when time allows

Intern
> Doer
> Patient's primary physician
> Learning to transition from doer to thinker
> Work closely with students in management of shared pts
> Not really expected to do any formal teaching

Student
> Follows 2-4 patients
> Acts as the primary provider with intern as backup
> Researches patient's medical problems in detail
> Correlates book knowledge with clinical care
> Spends time talking to patient

Pharm D
> Imbedded expert on all pharmacy related issues
> Will monitor appropriate use of medications
> Education of team and patients

Personal goals while on wards (be specific)

1.
2.
3.

Figure 4.2 Continued

liked or wanted to avoid? That led to a team discussion and a temporary consensus which might be adjusted over time with feedback from team members. "We've modified the plan over the last week and a half or so," a senior resident said, "to our own little version of what works best." Another attending seeks out personal details by inquiring about each individual's proudest moment and what they enjoy outside of the hospital's walls. After receiving feedback from a medical student about the desire to address issues of harassment and discrimination on the wards, one attending begins each new rotation with a dedicated conversation about how to prepare for, respond to, and debrief after instances of patient-initiated inappropriate behavior as a team, explicitly discussing how the team will commit to supporting each other when faced with challenging interactions.

These interactions with learners, particularly when discussing the learners' goals and clinical performance, were noticed and appreciated. One current learner commented that, "having that meeting or that feedback session in the beginning . . . showing that she is actually paying attention to you, wanting to improve week by week, is a big sign that she cares." And a former learner: "She would follow you where you were going and then identify deficits and scaffold knowledge on top of deficits, basically. She would support you where your goals were."

Using Learners' Names

Some attendings make it a point to memorize the names of the team members the night before that first meeting. At the session itself, they make sure they are pronouncing the names correctly. One current intern reported, with amazement, that his attending actually got his name right—something few other attendings had bothered to master. Also, starting with the first meeting, the attendings make liberal use of the first-person plural in referring to team activities. They say, "Why do *we* care?" It's "we"—not "you"—need to provide superb care for patients. Such small, tactful strategies go a long way toward creating a relaxed and collegial atmosphere.

Building the Team Through Personalization

Their personal styles and tastes dictate how the 18 attendings seek to put their teams at ease. One of them starts table rounds by playing recorded music. On the day we visited, the attending selected Tom Petty's "The Waiting" because one of the team's interns was awaiting the birth of his first child. There was banter back and forth about The Eagles band, and it was very clear that team members were comfortable with the attending and with each other. It was also obvious that the attending knew what was going on in the members' personal lives as well as in their clinical lives.

Attendings Develop Trust Through Balance

As the coach, the attending guides and corrects learners in ways that will maintain their ability to learn, do their work, and protect team cohesion. We will describe some of those specifics in the next few chapters. But the single most important factor, the cement that holds a team together, is the members' trust in each other and in their attending physician. The development of that mutual trust is one of the 18 attendings' major goals. A current learner, for example, told us that his attending had primed the pump from the start: "You feel that he comes into the team trusting that you know what you are doing and that you care about your patients. You don't want to lose that."

An important facet of any healthcare training experience is the balance between supervision and autonomy. The tightrope every teaching attending must walk involves ensuring that the learners gradually progress toward independent practice while consistently providing appropriate guidance and steering when wanted or needed. One current learner described this effective attending balancing act by stating, "She makes you think of your own decisions, run the team as a resident, but you know that you have her support and that she is always in the background."

This autonomy–supervision spectrum can be witnessed when the team discusses the plan of care with the patients. On some teams, the student or resident is asked to take the lead in facilitating discussion with the patients and their loved ones. This is not a decision made lightly. Hospitalized patients are often hungry for the most up-to-date information, including results of diagnostic tests, treatment plans, and discharge recommendations. To entrust a learner with communicating this critical information is a high form of autonomy indeed. Yet some attendings feel this is a key way to observe the learners' interpersonal skills—for instance, whether or not they avoid overly complex medical jargon when they share information—and the rapport they have built with their patients. A former learner said this of his attending:

> The one thing that stands out is the level of autonomy that I think she grants to all levels of learners, medical student through resident. One specific way in which that is expressed, I think, is—oftentimes going into the patient room—she will encourage the student or the residents to take the lead on the conversation rather than her, as the attending, to walk through whatever new information the team has developed or the plan for that day with any additional support as necessary. But she really kind of pushes for that autonomy from the very start.

Within other teams, it is the attending physician who takes the lead in discussing the plan of care with the patient. Attendings, often the team members with the most experience, are well positioned to field questions and role-model outstanding communication strategies. Indeed, multiple of the 18 attendings took the lead in the patients' rooms and did so with clarity and compassion. And, on some teams, there is a hybrid approach in which the attending leads conversations in the patient's room on some days of the rotation and learners lead conversations on others. This allows the attending to demonstrate effective communication while also providing opportunity for direct observation of and feedback on learners' communication skills.

Our attendings foster trust by demonstrating, day after day, that they commit to making sure the team's patients suffer no harm while, at the same time, giving team members the greatest possible freedom to diagnose and treat those patients. They also build trust by creating a supportive environment, a place where team members feel safe to make a mistake and call for help. How they go about it is the subject of the next chapter. First, though, a look at how the 18 attendings work with nurses, pharmacists, radiologists, and other hospital personnel.

Attendings Ensure Collaboration with All Team Members

The resident and the pharmacist were talking in the hall outside a patient's room; the attending physician was still inside the room. At a crucial moment, the pharmacist had come up with some information about the patient that the resident needed.

Resident (quietly, to pharmacist): "Thanks for bailing me out."
Pharmacist: "No problem. Anytime."
Attending: "I heard that!"
(Laughter all around.)

For most teaching settings, this would not be a typical encounter. According to a report summarizing the findings of a conference on the state of clinical education in the United States, "In most teaching settings, physicians learn and practice *alongside* nurses and other professionals rather than *with* them."[11] That was not what we saw in our observations of the 18 attendings who treated other hospital personnel as ex officio members of their teams, "instead of having them just do our work," as one current learner put it. When a patient's nurse was nearby and not otherwise occupied, they invited the nurse to join in the discussion on rounds. When pharmacists were part of rounds, their advice was sought, and they were included in the team camaraderie.

The "hidden curriculum," a phrase commonly used in medical education, describes "the processes, pressures and constraints which fall outside . . . the formal curriculum, and which are often unarticulated or unexplored."[12] It is this hidden curriculum, including attendings' behaviors toward others on the interprofessional team, that so often influences the behaviors (not to mention respect, demeanor, and outlook) of all team members. Attendings are watched and listened to closely. And they are emulated.

The attendings often led the team on forays to the radiology department, asking personnel there to go over the radiographic findings from a recent study and share their own pearls of wisdom. In these encounters, our attendings were invariably attentive and respectful. As one of them told us, "I don't want the team to think that anything I have to say is more valuable than what our pharmacist or the nurses have to say." The attendings wanted the information these personnel could give the team, but they were also acting in their capacity as role models. Physicians, they were indicating, should treat all providers as colleagues, both because it's the proper and respectful thing to do and because it can help the physician perform more efficiently. A failure of communication, so often the result of poor or nonexistent relationships, is a major cause of preventable, hospital-based error.[13] And, from the attending's personal point of view, patronizing or otherwise putting down colleagues is an effective formula for failure. Instead, the attendings we observed made it a point to foster connections with other colleagues, like one who was interacting with a palliative care fellow helping in the management of one of the team's patients. "You [the palliative care team] did a great job with the patient and his family. And I learned a few things from you."

We tagged along on a team visit to the radiology department. A resident radiologist pulled up the patient's images, and the team studied the film as the attending raised questions about it. The patient's images were then discussed by the attending radiologist, who was happy to show the team members some of the key elements in the film that pointed to a particular diagnosis. The group learned together in a collaborative and collegial environment, all facilitated by the attending.

We listened as an attending engaged a patient's bedside nurse, who had joined rounds and provided some helpful information to the team already.

Attending (to nurse): "Thank you. What else should we know to take good care of this patient today?"

Nurse: "I heard you wanted to give potassium. If you want that med to be given, I don't have an order for it."

Attending: "Great point."

(Attending then turned to the learner): "As we see the next patient, could you work with our RN colleague to ensure the medication order is entered and correct? I would appreciate it."

Throughout the entire encounter, the attending showed the nurse respect as a fellow professional provider and as a person. Thanking her and praising her behavior in front of the team was the right thing to do, but also served to strengthen the nurse's relationship with the group. By building positive connections with hospital personnel, the attendings find a particularly warm welcome when they take their teams to consult with those personnel.

Patients whose primary language is not concordant with physicians and other healthcare team members have disparate health outcomes, like poorer access to care, lower comprehension and satisfaction, and higher rates of complications.[14] Luckily, professional interpreters essentially erase these disparities and ensure that all patients, not just those with English proficiency, receive high-quality care.[14,15] One of our great attendings, while preparing to see the next patient, role-modeled appreciation for interpreters and imparted some learned wisdom to her team members: "Here are some things to remember that [the interpreter service] taught me. First, it's 'interpreter,' not 'translator.' Second, their role is to melt away so that we can have a discussion with the patient, not a discussion with the interpreter." And when the interpreter arrived, she did exactly that, with the attending holding the patient's hand and continuing consistent eye contact throughout the conversation, all with the interpreter in the background helping to bridge the language gap.

To get the most out of what a former learner calls "interdisciplinary pit stops," one of the attendings has her team figure out what information that particular specialist will need. This tactic is, in fact, a teaching tool that prompts learners to anticipate next steps in the patient's care plan, a concept we return to in a future chapter. It's also another way to demonstrate respect for other healthcare team members' time and to ensure the conversation stays focused on education rather than logistical details. The former learner offered some examples.

> If we want to consult nephrology for [acute kidney injury], what are they going to ask for? Are they going to ask for an ultrasound, are they going to ask for a urine study? Or if we were consulting neurology and we knew they were going to want a head MRI, we want to get that MRI done before we consult them. That way, it's more useful for them, and they can be ready for the next step.

In the next chapter, we show how our 18 attending physicians go about creating a supportive environment, one in which team members feel secure enough to accept and even welcome critical feedback as a necessary part of their path toward practice.

Main Points

1. The attendings use multiple strategies to build and maintain team relationships, such as acting as coaches, allowing learners to take the lead, entrusting team members in the care of their patients while providing necessary oversight, and getting to know each team member personally.
2. The attendings' definition of the team extends beyond learners and includes all members of the interprofessional health-care team.
3. Attendings view the care of a patient as the team's responsibility and not just that of the intern.

Further Reading

Cooke M, Irby DM, Sullivan W, Ludmerer KM. American medical education 100 years after the Flexner Report. N Engl J Med 2006;355:1339–44.

In this article, the authors summarize the changes in medical education over the past century and describe current challenges. Medical knowledge has vastly expanded, while delivery of care has also become more complicated. The authors call for the use of various knowledge assessments to ensure that professional values, medical knowledge, and skills are attained.

Finn KM, Metlay JP, Chang Y, et al. Effect of increased inpatient attending physician supervision on medical errors, patient safety, and resident education: A randomized clinical trial. JAMA Intern Med 2018;178:952–9.

The role of attending physician supervision on patient safety was evaluated in this 9-month randomized clinical trial. Performed on an inpatient general medicine unit in a large academic medical center, 22 attending physicians provided standard or increased levels of supervision on patient care rounds. More than 1,200 patients were included in the analysis. Results showed no significant difference on the rate of medical error between the two groups. However, interns reported feeling less efficient and less autonomous with an attending physician present, underscoring the importance of effective supervision–autonomy balance.

Manojlovich M, Harrod M, Hofer TP, Lafferty M, McBratnie M, Krein SL. Using qualitative methods to explore communication practices in the context of patient care rounds on general care units. J Gen Intern Med 2020;35:839–45.

Prior studies have shown that poor communication between physicians and nurses is a contributor to adverse events for hospitalized patients. In this qualitative study, 163 physicians and nurses at four Midwest hospitals were observed with the purpose of better understanding communication practices. Direct observations, focus groups, and interviews were all conducted. Based on the gathered data, communication was broken down into three contextual dimensions: organizational complexity (driven by workflow differences), cognitive load of clinicians, and social context. The results suggest that organizations seeking to improve communication should consider the complexity of communication and the context in which it occurs.

5

A Safe, Supportive Environment

I never teach my pupils, I only attempt to provide the conditions in which they can learn.

—Albert Einstein

In the previous chapter, we described team learning as "knowledge gained through participation in a dynamic community of practice." Once an attending has started to build the team and foster trusting relationships among its members, the next goal is to cultivate the dynamic nature of this community of practice through true collaboration. Our 18 outstanding teaching physicians achieve that team-oriented goal, in part, by creating a climate in which learners feel it is safe to answer a question incorrectly and to debate with their attending. Learners discover that they and their ideas are valued and that their mistakes are treated as learning opportunities—for themselves and other team members.

This view of clinical education is a far cry from that experienced by learners of earlier generations (and by many learners still today) in which the attendings were seen as the ultimate authority and could not be questioned. Too often, attending physicians on ward rounds lecture more than they listen, instruct more than they inquire. In our interviews of current and former learners, some spoke of being criticized or demeaned by different attending physicians in front of others. As a current learner suggested, the impact can be lasting: "I think the first time you get shot down by an attending on rounds, especially like the first day or something, you're not going to

Teaching Inpatient Medicine. Second Edition. Nathan Houchens, Molly Harrod, and Sanjay Saint, Oxford University Press. © Nathan Houchens, Molly Harrod, and Sanjay Saint 2023. DOI: 10.1093/oso/9780197639023.003.0005

say much more to that person for a while. Probably not going to have the courage."

That result is precisely what the 18 attendings strive to prevent. Embarrassment, anxiety, and fear are enemies of rational, creative thinking and the learning process. A substantial body of research supports the view that the most effective clinical education is collaborative rather than command and control, experiential rather than through rote memorization and passive lectures.[1]

Our attendings are able to create collaborative, experiential learning environments by continuing to build relationships with individual team members and by providing support when learners encounter challenges or uncertainties—be they systemic, professional, or personal. Additionally, attendings seek to gain learners' trust, in part through mutual trust to fulfill their respective roles on the team. Finally, attendings acquire a sense of the needs and goals of individual team members and strive to meet them. In other words, coupled with their extensive knowledge base, clinical acumen, and expertise in the field, the best teaching attendings harness substantial people skills to create and sustain a safe, supportive learning environment. As a review of the literature concerning the attributes of excellent clinical teachers suggests, success as an attending "depends less on the acquisition of cognitive skills such as medical knowledge and formulating learning objectives, and more on inherent, relationship-based, non-cognitive attributes."[2]

Such interactional behaviors may come naturally to some, while for others, it requires intense effort. Fortunately, these behaviors and techniques are collectively known as *people skills*, and like other skills, they can be learned, practiced, and improved upon. In this chapter, we consider the approaches that the 18 outstanding attending physicians use to make team members feel safe and supported while learning to practice clinical inpatient medicine.

Positive, Welcoming Communication Styles

The behavior of the attendings toward team members and other hospital personnel establishes an environment that is warm, welcoming, and accepting. As both current and former learners told us with re-markable consistency, and as we witnessed directly, the attendings were generous with their praise for all team members, which helped to create a positive atmosphere within the team. Sometimes the attendings' approval was expressed with a simple elbow bump or a thumbs up, and sometimes with the simplest of words: "Great job," "Nice work," "Way to go," "That's exactly what I would do."

We witnessed the following exchange between one of our attendings and a resident:

Attending: I thought you were going to get there. I was trying to lead you there.
Resident: I know. [They high-five.]
Attending: I like how proud you make me. It makes my heart warm.

The attendings' speech patterns and body language reinforce a sup-portive environment. Most of them speak calmly and quietly. They are part of the circle of team members during rounds, positioned alongside (rather than in front of) their team members. Some make it a point to ask the person presenting to speak to all team members rather than focus their attention on the attending. As one of the attendings described his participation on rounds: "It takes us three or four days at the beginning of the month for people to understand to stop looking at me."

Attendings' eyes remained on the presenter, listening carefully and respectfully (see Figure 5.1). They rarely interrupted presentations, holding off any comments until the learner had completed their thoughts; if seriously critical comments were necessary, they were generally delayed until they could be made to the presenter in pri-vate. On those occasions when the attendings did interrupt, it was to seek clarification, and it was done apologetically.

In their interactions with learners outside of rounds, the attendings present themselves as open and accessible, easy to re-late to and talk with. They smile and maintain eye contact. There is no sense of impatience, no suggestion that they need to move on to other priorities. They are fully present with their learners and treat

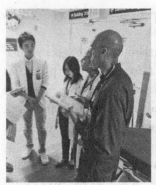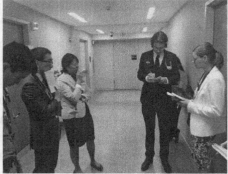

Figure 5.1 Senior residents leading rounds with the attendings listening in.

them as colleagues. "When he's there, he's there," a learner said, "so there's nothing else on his mind."

The attendings also cultivate meaningful relationships with their learners, engaging them in conversations about their interests and activities outside the hospital. One of the attendings described his approach: "I say, 'Where are you from? Where did you go to high school? What did you do after college?' Invariably, the stories are great. You know, people have done amazing things." In another instance, as learners gathered in the team room for rounds, we witnessed one attending ask her intern, "How was wine and cheese last night?" It was clear that she knew much about the learner's current life outside of the hospital and cared to inquire about it.

Available and Eager to Help

The attendings make it clear that they are ready and eager to assist their team members when problems arise, day or night. On one level, that is the basic, all-important habit attendings request of their learners: contact me when you want or need to discuss an important aspect of the patient's care, when you are feeling uncomfortable, or when you are not sure what to do. The knowledge that the attending is there for them comforts and at least partially relieves learners of the fear of mistakes that could worsen a patient's condition or cost a patient their life.

Our 18 attendings make sure their teams know how to get in touch with them 24 hours a day, 7 days a week. A former learner put it this way: "You can call him at 8 PM and he won't be pissed. He's like, 'Call me any time you have a problem; I'm ready to come on in and work it out with you.'" Many of the physicians rearrange their schedules for the time when they would be serving as teaching attending, as some have recommended.[3] "I try to decrease to only absolutely urgent meetings for these 2 weeks," an attending told us, "so I'm not distracted and can be available for them if needed." It's a crucial element to convey a safe and supportive environment.

On another level, the 18 attendings also make themselves available to help with nonclinical problems or concerns that are unique to individual team members. Sometimes, learners sought their advice about family challenges or even money troubles. "I still go to her for advice about personal things and work things," a former learner said. Frequent requests from learners included guidance about their career paths, help coping with what one learner called "hospital systems issues," trouble getting through to a particular physician, or arranging for a diagnostic test in a reasonable time frame. The attendings may be able to cut through the red tape and get the task accomplished more quickly.

At various points during the day, our attendings usually check in with the team, by text or in person, and they sometimes make a late afternoon or nightly call to see if help is needed. If it is a particularly hectic time, they may volunteer to talk with a patient's loved ones, write some progress notes, or even temporarily take over a few patients so that an overwhelmed learner can complete their clinical responsibilities on time.

Invest in Learners and the Team

The 18 attendings do not simply make themselves physically available; they are also alert for situations in which they can tailor the learning experience to the individual. At table rounds, they make sure to include extra material in their discussions that would be of interest to particular team members. "I will be certain to mention visceral and cutaneous leishmaniasis," one of the attendings told us, "because they are endemic in the part of the world the intern is from." We heard another attending urging two medical students to view an interventional radiology procedure involving the abdomen because "GI is your thing." He even had a handout on the procedure to share with them.

A former learner recalled that, when she was an intern, she was intensely worried about her lack of knowledge of intravenous catheters; she did not, for example, know the difference between a central line and a dialysis catheter. When she mentioned this to her attending, she "sat me down and got out a catheter and took something that I was especially concerned about and really made it easy for me."

In another example, the attending was creating a teaching moment on rounds by facilitating discussion around the differences between aspiration pneumonitis and aspiration pneumonia in elderly patients and those with neurologic conditions. The team had a learner whose future career involved neurology, so the attending turned her attention to that learner, saying, "you'll see this situation a lot on neurology." And later, she harnessed that learner's enthusiasm for neurologic topics by asking, "Did you notice how he grabbed my hand? That's a frontal release sign. Do you want to demonstrate that?"

The attendings understand that a word of support and empathy can have a great impact. When a student was asked a question by the senior resident about choice and duration of antibiotics for a complicated patient, the attending normalized the difficulty by briefly and quietly interjecting to the student, "That's a tough one." In another example, a learner told us about one of his patients who was suffering with chronic pain and depression. The team had enlisted the help of the acute pain service, but the pain specialists had unexpectedly signed off, saying they had done everything they could. "It put us in this position of, we're general medicine," the learner recalled. "What can *we* do?" The learner called her attending that night to provide an update and told her about the patient. " 'This sucks,' is basically what [the attending] said," the learner reported, "and she said, 'They put you in a bad situation and that's really frustrating. You're doing everything that you can.' And so, it was nice. It was like she sort of reinforced what we were trying to do."

Our 18 attendings invest in their learners and want them to succeed throughout their training—attitudes that their learners recognize and draw comfort from. This comment by one of the attendings makes the point:

> Oftentimes, I ask for July or August because I really love the newbies. I love when they're new and kind of excited. But I also feel really compelled to kind of set the stage, set expectations, help them kind of get a really good start on what it means to provide good inpatient care. Sometimes, if you don't get a good start right off the bat, then you kind of go down the other end. So, I feel a real responsibility.

The attendings consider themselves lifelong learners, right alongside other members of the team. Learners acknowledged feeling more engaged when they realized how much their attendings enjoyed teaching and how much these world-class physicians wanted to keep learning. "He's still just, you know, very enthusiastic about what he is teaching," a current learner told us. "And very curious—very much there to discover new things along with you." That frame of mind, universal among the 18 attendings, helps create a probing, intellectually stimulating climate that serves both the team and patients.

Push with Positivity

From their first encounters with a new team, these attendings clearly lay out their expectations regarding learners' roles and responsibilities. Individual goals are set for the medical students, the interns, and the residents, including what they can and should attain during their weeks on the wards. The 18 attendings tend to set the bar high. A current learner described for us how his attending furthered those expectations.

> You can tell you're being pushed to do what you're capable of, but you're being pushed with positivity and like, "Hey, I think you can do this for your patient. I think you're good enough to really take ownership and be the primary manager for this patient's care." It's a very supportive and positive way of getting you to put yourself out there and push yourself to your limits.

Our attendings generally give learners autonomy in their clinical decision-making. We heard about several instances in which the attending had one plan in mind while the learner had proposed an alternative approach. If the learner's plan was not going to harm the patient or delay care, the attending approved of its implementation. A current learner spoke of his experience with one of the 18 attendings.

> I have had attendings where minor things like pain medicines or minor things like just doses of the same medicine, they would not want you to even experiment with doses. They want their dose and that's what they want. [Our current attending] was like, "Yeah, sure. You think that's going to work? Just do it. Try it. Make sure you have enough safeguards around that you won't end up killing the patient but try it. And if it doesn't work, great. Come back to what I am saying or, if it works, even better! I will learn from you!"

From a learner's perspective, the freedom to make independent patient care decisions is probably the most important demonstration of the attendings' support and trust. Of course, this autonomy is only made possible because of the layers of protection provided by the attending, the senior resident, and the consulting providers. This is where the rubber meets the road, where learners develop the clinical skills and the self-assurance to become practicing physicians. As one of the attendings tells her teams, "My job is to protect you from making a mistake that will wipe away your confidence." In a note-worthy example, when a learner was getting paged to leave rounds and evaluate a deteriorating patient, they quickly went through their diagnostic thought process with the attending, to which the attending responded, "Thanks for the heads up. I know you have a good plan."

A former learner recalled a moment when her attending urged her to take the lead in a difficult conversation with a patient. It was a challenging assignment, but the learner felt "completely comfortable," she said, "knowing that the attending was there in a supportive role if I had any kind of questions. And she really sat back and let me take the lead." The learner recognized that it might have been much easier for the attending to just have the conversation herself. "I'm toward the end of residency now," the learner said. "I'm realizing how valuable those experiences are in preparing me for future practice." The time learners spend leading conversations or bedside presentations also serves to prepare them for another kind of future activity—as teachers, as attending physicians.

The Spirit of Learning Together

In pursuit of the best possible care for their patients, some attendings insisted that team members not automatically accept the attending's diagnostic or treatment proposals. If a learner has a different view, they are encouraged to challenge the attending.

We witnessed an exchange between a medical student and one of our attendings. When the attending disagreed with the learner's assessment of a patient's symptom, the learner responded, "Oh, okay." The attending quickly responded, "Don't just melt away. I expect push-back." Another attending put it this way, when discussing with a learner who reported a cardiac murmur while listening to a patient's heart (that the attending had not heard): "Stick to your guns. If you really hear it the way you heard it, make sure you don't give up on that." The goal of this "put your nickel down" approach is twofold: to foster independent thinking and to encourage team members to advocate for their patients and themselves. Such independent thinking is necessary, as our attendings are well aware, because they are fallible. They do not have all the answers. A former learner remembered an example.

There have been times when he has asked question, question, question. Nobody knows, and then he admits that he doesn't know either. So, everybody goes and looks it up. So, it's that level of informality. The whole thing turns out to be a fun learning experience.

Another moment of humility arose when a night resident was presenting a patient to the team. The resident's plan was to ease the patient's itching with a medicine that would treat elevated bilirubin levels. The attending commented, "I actually didn't know that," to the resident and then, to the team's pharmacist, "Do you know how that works?"

Some attendings are also quick to admit their errors and gaps in knowledge. "When I make a mistake, I tell them," one reported. "I say, 'That's exactly what you don't want to do, is just what I did in there. Remember that. Don't ever do that.'" Each of the attendings has a store of personal mistakes that they might draw upon when relevant; they recognize that failure is a most valuable teaching opportunity. Likewise, our attendings are keen to admit that they don't always know the answer. As a resident was describing their decision on when to use a particular invasive medical device, the attending commented with a shrug, "I'll take your word for it because I have no idea."

While rounding, we heard the following exchange between an attending and his team member:

Intern: The patient's blood pressure has decreased since we started the medication.

Attending: [High-fiving the senior resident] You were right! I said it wouldn't go down, but you said to wait and see and you were right. I owe you one.

The willingness on the part of some attendings to admit ignorance or error has another important effect. It seems to contribute to the creation of a safe environment for learners by presenting mistakes as natural and inevitable aspects of the clinical learning process. If attendings are comfortable with and able to air their limitations, it becomes easier for learners to accept their own without fear of embarrassment. A former learner summarized this concept succinctly, noting, "You need to make people feel comfortable about putting their thoughts out so that you can actually say no or yes and correct them, and if you make them comfortable saying that, they will come up with more questions that will trigger a good learning environment."

It is important to note that the practices of admitting one's mistakes and demonstrating fallibility are not universally adopted by all teaching attendings in their teams. Particularly among those attendings who are early in their careers and those who identify as female or as an underrepresented minority in medicine, these behaviors are less commonly used and, in fact, sometimes specifically and purposefully avoided. Rather, some attendings feel the need to assert themselves consistently and confidently with their teams and at the bedside. This need arises, as we noted in a previous chapter, because of comments from patients, their family members, and other providers that indicate the attendings are not recognized as leaders, not qualified for their roles, and sometimes mistaken for other members of the healthcare team. Likewise, at times, others may question the attendings' thought processes and decisions simply because of who they are as people. One former learner commented, "I can see [female attendings] have to talk a little bit louder . . . they have to be a little bit more, not forceful, but more direct about patient care issues." This is an important reminder that the strategies and techniques used by one outstanding teaching attending may not be broadly applicable to all.

Mistakes Are Opportunities

In instances when the learner's suggested approach does not go according to plan, the attendings look for a way to move forward without embarrassing the learner or diminishing the learner's confidence and relationship with the patient. They seek to personify the quote from Nelson Mandela: "I never lose. I either win or learn." Here's an example as told to us by a current learner.

> At no point did she [the attending] throw me under the bus or make the patient feel that way. I think she just sort of said, "We've done exactly what we said we were going to do. We discussed this plan of controlling your pain, and now we're going to move to the alternative form of treatment which is what you want." And I think that made the patient happy, and it made me not feel like I was marginalized or disrespected in any way.

In that way, the attending makes it possible for the learner to continue their management of the patient—and their education—in a positive frame of mind. Contrast that with the negative feelings of an errant learner who is embarrassed or even ridiculed in front of other team members. Learning flourishes best in a safe, supportive environment.

To that end, the 18 attending physicians strongly believe in positive feedback that reinforces effective behaviors. On rounds, we heard one attending say to the team, "[The medical student] has really been working to streamline his presentations, and it shows!" Conversely, correction in the clinical setting, they believe, needs to be very different from that in a typical classroom. An attending explained: "I need to be able to tell them what they need to do better without them interpreting that as me giving them a grade."

Our attendings avoid the word "wrong" like the plague. Instead, they follow a core principle of improvisation:[4] they build on the learner's thought processes by saying "Yes, and. . . ." Again and again, learners told us that the correction process is not judgmental, that it never feels demeaning or condescending. When a learner makes a mistake, attendings engage them in a discussion, often asking questions to find out what led to the incorrect conclusion. A former learner offered an extreme example: "You could say, 'I think this patient is sick because there was an alien invasion last night.' He would be, like, 'That's really a great idea, and what do you think about this?'"

In medicine, there are all kinds of mistakes that a learner can make, of course, starting with the simple inability to answer a question. The 18 attendings generally start their questioning with the medical students on the team, geared to their knowledge level and often focused on clinical reasoning rather than rote recall. If a learner seems to be having difficulty with a question or comes up with an incorrect answer, the attendings generally redirect the question to another learner, with or without comment. A current learner told us about making a wrong suggestion and what his attending had to say about it.

> So, he was like, "No, no, it's okay. You probably said this because you figured this thing, which is a good thought process, but in this case, it's not really applicable because of this thing." So that made me feel okay. I wasn't as stupid as I might have sounded. So, that is, I think, very, very important. I mean, it keeps you going.

When one of our attendings gives a learner feedback after a presentation and in front of other team members, the attending does so in a manner to avoid upsetting the presenter. Here is a feedback sample we observed: "Excellent presentation. Good job! I want to talk about [the patient] medically. You didn't say this, but I saw in his chart that he had not been able to lie flat in two years." And another: "Excellent, you gave us all the essential stuff. You have to remember he came to us for chest discomfort, so you gave us a bit too much on his psychiatric and family history. Write it in the medical record, but you can omit most of it for your oral presentation." And finally: "Very well organized. Nice succinct story. Most remarkable was his systolic blood pressure of 90. You mentioned stopping his fluids . . . is his blood pressure back to normal?"

If there is an error in patient care, our attendings' first reaction is to determine how and why it happened, and what effect it might have on the learner's performance. They are curious rather than accusatory. A former learner described that kind of encounter.

> He would stop and say, "Just a second. What happened?" You know, before blaming him, saying, "Oh, that person is terrible. . . ." And he gives so much credit to everyone, in terms of trying to understand what were the circumstances, why this happened.

Attending Emotions

A number of our exemplary attendings demonstrate remarkable emotional intelligence. Emotional intelligence has been described as "the ability to understand your own emotions and those of other people and to use that knowledge to change the way you behave toward them."[5,6] Rather than a simple intuition of how others feel, harnessing emotional intelligence requires considerable introspection to understand one's personal emotions and how to handle them in social contexts. Fortunately, this means emotional intelligence can improve, depending on the amount of time and energy invested.

Several attendings demonstrated use of emotional intelligence to motivate and change learners' behavior. On rare occasions, anger from an attending may surface—especially when learners are shirking their responsibilities and accountability. If the attending has invested in the team member, built that relationship, and clearly conveyed high expectations, anger and frustration may serve as an important communication tool when something is amiss, just as a coach might demonstrate these emotions with an athlete. "I come down hard on them," one attending told us, "if the mistake they make is out of laziness or inattentiveness or not checking something. A couple of residents here have a very cavalier attitude, and that really frustrates me!"

Another attending was exasperated when she reviewed a learner's progress note concerning a patient who had come in the night before with dizziness, which requires a thorough history. Yet the learner's written history appeared to be very similar to that from the emergency department provider, and he told the same story in the same way on rounds. It wasn't the first time the learner had cut corners, so the attending walked the learner into the patient's room, and they took the patient's history together. "We had a conversation," the attending told us, "and I said [to the learner], 'I think you're a better physician than what you're showing me.'"

Far more evident than anger in the 18 attendings' arsenal is their sense of humor, which serves as a key ingredient in relieving tensions and creating a safe and supportive environment (see Figure 5.2). "Half of his communication is through humor," a current learner told us, "so it makes . . . rounding very comfortable." The humor may take the form of self-deprecation, although it is sometimes aimed at the learners as well. "Because he is able to make fun of himself in

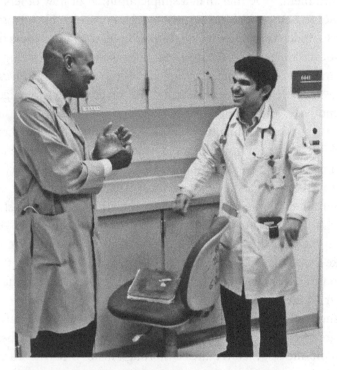

Figure 5.2 Attending and learner joking during rounds.

front of us," another current learner added, "when he teases other people, it doesn't seem like it's done in a mean-spirited way." Just as before, some attendings view self-deprecation as a luxury that they cannot or should not employ because of who they are and because of the need to consistently reinforce their role as team lead.

The jokes generally emerge out of a given situation as the attending and team conduct rounds. Here is one we watched develop. An attending spotted some written marks on the back of a patient's hand. "What's this?" he asked. "Something real important," the patient responded. "Oh," said the attending, "I thought you went clubbing last night."

Humor is a time-honored technique of establishing rapport with people in general, and it also serves that function within a clinical team. We heard one of our attendings as she was reviewing and pointing out anatomical features of the different types of intestine on abdominal radiographs with the team. "[Pointing] What is this, large bowel or small bowel?" And while awaiting a response from the team, "See, the clue here is the big red arrow."

In the next two chapters, we focus less on the people skills of the 18 attendings and more on their day-to-day teaching tools and techniques. The topics vary greatly, from a cure for a blank look to the uses of mnemonics, whiteboards, and smartphones, but they have in common that they were used successfully by some terrific clinician-educators.

Main Points

1. The 18 attendings all create a safe and supportive learning environment but use various strategies to do so, such as supporting team members in both their professional and personal lives, being clear in their high expectations of learners, seeking to understand errors rather than admonishing, and using emotion to communicate and stimulate learning.

2. The attendings provide positive, reinforcing feedback and are completely engaged during rounds. They make themselves

available to learners and are eager to help in a myriad of ways. The attendings also get to know the learners on a personal level in order to build trusting relationships.

3. Some, though not all, attendings admit their own mistakes and welcome challenges from learners, demonstrating the conviction that a mistake is a prime learning opportunity. Learners engage in clinical decision-making knowing that their attending will support and protect them in case of an oversight.

Further Reading

Kelly E, Richards JB. Medical education: giving feedback to doctors in training. BMJ 2019;366:l4523.

Providing feedback is an essential component of any teaching activity. This article explores the various ways in which feedback can and should be given while teaching. Feedback is a crucial component of reflection and constructive skills modification—and not just for those learning a new skill. With a lack of existing international guidelines, this paper examines the extant literature to synthesize a collection of specific characteristics of effective feedback. The overall process the authors elucidate here involves clarifying to teachers why feedback is important for learners, ensuring the focus of the feedback is to empower learners, finding the appropriate space and time to give and receive feedback, and establishing a repeatable feedback process. Feedback provided to learners needs to be specific, relevant, and focused on objective behaviors.

Savage BM, Lujan HL, Thipparthi RR, DiCarlo SE. Humor, laughter, learning, and health! A brief review. Adv Physiol Educ 2017;41:341–7.

In this in-depth piece, the authors delve into the history and impact of humor and health. Properly used, humor can help relieve stress (by reducing the amount of cortisol and epinephrine in a person's system) and, in doing so, it creates a protected space where learning can occur. Documenting the rich, anecdotal history of salutatory effects of humor on health, this treatise examines the intersection of the mind, body, and emotions. With a detailed examination of the evidence gathered on the topic in recent decades, this paper makes a compelling argument for the benefits of properly used humor in the healthcare setting. Many readers may be familiar with Hunter "Patch" Adams—a physician immortalized on the big screen by the late, great Robin Williams—who conceptualized healing as an act of love, not transaction, between physician and patient. Dr. Adams frequently used humor (in the form of therapeutic hospital clowns) as a tool to help patients heal. In sum, this article tells the tale of the many ways in which humor can help everyone live a better, healthier, and more learned life.

Carbo AR, Huang GC. Promoting clinical autonomy in medical learners. Clin Teach 2019;16:454–7.

In this practical guide, the authors discuss a set of teachers' tools to help their learners develop a critical skill in medicine: clinical autonomy. In this context, the authors define clinical autonomy as "being able to act of one's volition," and this article provides specific, actionable steps teachers can take to foster clinical autonomy in their trainees. These steps include a needs assessment by the teacher on the first day with new trainees, gently pushing trainees to the edge of—and then beyond—their comfort zone, prompting trainees to delineate their thinking process concerning specific decisions (e.g., obtaining an ultrasound before a CT), and understanding when to step in for the best interests of the patient (and when to step out to allow trainees to grow). By following these steps, teachers can provide space both for their supervision and for trainee autonomy, and these guidelines can and should be modified for local healthcare culture.

6

Bedside and Beyond

The good physician treats the disease; the great physician treats the patient who has the disease.

—William Osler

As the practice of medicine has become increasingly complex over the years, the clinical education of medical learners has inevitably become ever more complicated and demanding. There is so much new information to be conveyed, so many new treatments, so much new technology. At the same time, hours spent in training have been substantially reduced. These developments have whittled away at a centuries-old, essential aspect of clinical education: bedside teaching.

Well before the 2003 restriction of interns' duty hours, concerns were being raised over how little time learners were engaged in direct patient interaction; studies suggested that less than 25% of clinical teaching was taking place at the bedside.[1] And, in 2013, a team from Johns Hopkins discovered that interns were spending time at the bedside, examining and conversing with patients, only 12% of their work day, while more than 40% was spent in front of a computer.[2]

Some healthcare providers have recognized this threat to effective bedside teaching, learning, and connection. In 2017, a group of global physician educators (of which one of our outstanding attendings is a key leader) established the Society of Bedside Medicine, an organization "dedicated to bedside teaching and improving physical examination and diagnostic skills" whose purpose "is to foster a culture of bedside medicine through deliberate practice and teaching,

Teaching Inpatient Medicine. Second Edition. Nathan Houchens, Molly Harrod, and Sanjay Saint,
Oxford University Press. © Nathan Houchens, Molly Harrod, and Sanjay Saint 2023.
DOI: 10.1093/oso/9780197639023.003.0006

and by encouraging innovation in education and research on the role of the clinical encounter in 21st century medicine."[3] As another recent marker of efforts to enhance bedside teaching, in 2018, the Accreditation Council of Graduate Medical Education (ACGME) founded the "Back to Bedside" initiative, "designed to empower residents and fellows to develop transformative projects that foster meaning and joy in work and allow them to engage on a deeper level with what is at the heart of medicine: their patients."[4]

The 18 outstanding attending physicians we observed and interviewed were well aware of the pressures that are pulling learners away from the bedside. They join the chorus of voices from the ACGME, Society of Bedside Medicine, and others to resist this pull. The attendings are strong supporters and insistent practitioners of bedside teaching, determined to give their learners as much of it as possible. One of the attendings told us, "As we move toward shorter rounds and shorter time for our learners, more of the time we've been spending in [table] rounds and presenting has to be spent with the patient and the problem."

Structures and Strategies That Maximize Teaching Time

The 18 attendings we observed had their individual, unique instructional strategies and tactics. In this chapter, we discuss some of the various ways in which they go about their inspired teaching.

Our attendings share many attributes and attitudes. When we asked them to identify the primary goal of bedside teaching, for example, their answers were remarkably similar. "Providing not just random trivial facts," one replied, "but patient-applicable knowledge [that learners] can carry forward, taking it to the bedside of the next patient and figuring where it fits and where it doesn't fit." Another attending spoke of learners applying this knowledge "to make a good clinical decision," while a third cited the need to present the knowledge "in a way that people can remember." Thus, the role of the teaching attending is to facilitate learning in the context of the individual patient that can inform sound clinical decisions in a manner that learners remember and apply to future patients.

Effective time management is critical in modern inpatient rounds. By their very nature, patient rounds are not the ideal setting for the delivery of a full-scale teaching script on a particular symptom or disease. It steals too much time from the already limited time available for patient rounds. Instead, our attendings seek to anticipate teaching moments and prepare brief lessons that are relevant to the patients who will be seen on rounds. "Some attendings," a current learner lamented, "go on and on about things that aren't related to the patient, or they'll just talk too long. And once that happens, you start to space out and zone out." On the other hand, his attending, one of our outstanding 18, is "really good at finding teaching points, little pearls."

Attendings find ways to proactively adjust their schedules to the peaks and valleys of their learners' days. "She knew that there didn't have to be an hour of teaching every day if we were too busy," a current learner said of his attending. She also won the gratitude of her residents by having medical students deliver abbreviated presentations on team rounds, saving residents precious minutes for their other work. "I really appreciated that!" one of her residents exclaimed. The attending would ensure medical students received practice by listening to their full presentations during one-on-one meetings.

As part of the process of setting clear expectations for learners, attendings often communicate their preferences regarding the format oral patient presentations should take. A variety of abbreviated presentations exist. For instance, a traditional presentation structure on rounds is known as the "E-SOAP" presentation, which stands for Events, Subjective, Objective, Assessment, and Plan. It starts with the learner presenting the overnight and interval events, subjective concerns as relayed by the patient, objective findings on the physical examination (beginning with the vital signs) as well as all diagnostic tests and other results finalized since the previous day, and concludes with the assessment and plan, either by problem or by organ system.

To make rounds more efficient, some attendings choose to focus on just the events overnight and assessment and plan by problem (so-called EAP presentations). In this structure, if the patient had a fever overnight, fever would be listed as a problem to discuss. Any and all pertinent subjective reports; examination findings; diagnostic test results; and assessment and plan related to the fever would be discussed during that particular problem. And the process would repeat in an iterative fashion for each problem, such as low sodium, continued abdominal pain, or new-onset diarrhea.

There have been remarkably few examinations of preferences for different presentation structures. In one study, however, researchers surveyed learners (medical students and resident physicians), directly comparing their thoughts on EAP and SOAP formats, and the results were striking.[5] Among learners who had experience in delivering patient information in both formats, they tended to prefer EAP to SOAP. In particular, while they felt there was no difference in ease of use between structures, learners felt that use of EAP, compared with SOAP, better encouraged them to distill pertinent information; integrate information from the history, exam, and studies into the assessment and plan; and focus on the assessment and plan. Additionally, EAP was considered more time-efficient. While each attending has their preferred style, it appears that EAP resonates with how learners think.

One area in which the attendings differed in their approach was rounding structure. Some would see and examine every patient, with presentations delivered at the bedside; others asked for presentations outside the patient's room; and still others discussed patients around a table (table rounds). Many encouraged a hybrid of several of these strategies, and some noted that this structure changed day to day depending on the needs of and time pressures on the team. We witnessed one attending preparing with her team just before rounds: "Let's plan to stop rounds at 10:30 so that we have some teaching flexibility. I'd like [the senior resident] to prioritize patients we see together. We can do bedside rounds in the rooms for some of our patients." This was followed immediately by a discussion of how to effectively deliver an oral patient presentation in front of the patient. All attendings saw at least some patients with the team every day, and a common thread was that all types of rounds were thoughtfully executed through effective preparation.

The decision of which patients to see as a team and in which order of priority is often delegated to the senior resident. In fact, this is a teaching tool as well. It allows the attending to observe the thought processes and prioritization of the resident. One of the attendings reported: "I round on every patient every day, but I don't round on every patient with the team every day." That kind of arrangement, he said, allows them to give their full attention during bedside rounds, because it limits the team rounding time to two hours a day, and they do not have to worry about, as he put it, "Oh, my God! Am I ever going to get to put an order in?" A current learner told us of another accommodation made by one of the attendings. "If we don't see my patients as a [team]," the learner said, "he will come back and see them individually with me. I've never had anyone do that before." All of the attendings made it a point to see every patient assigned to their team every day, whether they were newly admitted patients or existing ones.

Teaching outside of rounds also comes with attending expectations. For example, one attending will show up at the team room on an afternoon to do some teaching targeted at medical students and will inform them that he wants their undivided attention. On the other hand, he tells the interns and residents in the team room— most of whom are furiously clacking away on the computer—that he only wants half of their attention. His empathy toward his learners comes through when he mentions, "It's just hard for busy residents and interns to say, 'Okay, I can give you my undivided attention for the next 20 minutes.'"

The Cornerstones of Clinical Medicine

Relationship-based communication with patients during the clinical interview, combined with an effective physical examination, are and always will be the cornerstones of clinical bedside medicine. As you might expect, the 18 attendings we observed are outstanding bedside teachers. To begin with, they are virtuoso clinicians and diagnosticians.

It may seem like the most basic and elementary of lessons an attending can teach their learners: if you want to find out what is happening with a patient, ask the patient. One form of such inquiry is the physical examination. Whether it's performed by a learner or an attending, the exam needs to be deliberate and thorough, using all senses to ask and answer questions about the patient's condition. The more obvious form of questioning is verbal: talk to the patient about their symptoms, feelings, and lived experiences.

The problem-oriented medical interview is a staple of traditional medical practice, though the invasion of new technologies and the ramped-up time and administrative pressures on attendings and learners threaten to dilute the clinical focus on the patient. A former learner described how his attending combats this trend: "Instead of just looking at what we know from lab studies or imaging or talking to consultants, he often asks patients what they first noticed when they were diagnosed with the condition . . . back to the original [concern]."

A current learner spoke of his attending's insistence on individualizing patient care by providing a holistic perspective. This involved appreciating what was best for the patient—not just in terms of which medicine would best alleviate the symptom or pro-long life, but also how to maximize quality of life and attend to the patient's priorities. One learner made the comparison of attendings who prioritize medicine to those who prioritize the patient. "A lot of times," he said, "attendings don't kind of talk to the patient as much. We don't kind of look at the whole situation of the patient when we make decisions. He does."

Teaching attendings listened closely to the patients. They recognized concerns, even if only briefly mentioned by patients, and made it a point to prioritize them for the patient's overall well-being. While making rounds with one of the 18 attendings, we saw two examples within an hour of his intense attention to his patients. The exchanges occurred after the team left the patients' rooms.

Attending: Time to critique the attending. Why did I question her about depression?

Intern: She started tearing up.

Attending: She said, "I feel bad." There's often a little window you get in the course of a conversation. The key is to follow that window. It's important to think about picking up and following those cues.

A short time later: another patient, another insight. The attending addressed the medical student.

Attending: So there was something we heard when we were leaving the bedside.

Medical student: Something about anxiety.

Attending [to intern]: That's something we should make her PCP [primary care provider] aware of.

Patients generally enter a hospital because of a single acute problem. "On a busy call day," a former learner told us, "we kind of tunnel our vision on this one big thing. But if you talk with the patients, there might be several other subacute or chronic problems. If there was anything significant going on with a patient, [our attending] required us to be on top of that. And it's not that it took a lot more time or energy to provide more holistic care for the patient instead of just focusing on one thing."

The bedside physical examination was stressed by the teaching attendings we observed and interviewed as a vital tool in the physician's toolbelt. One former learner described his attending: "His physical exam skills were amazing. He would often pick up on things just by looking at the patients. When he would notice something about the patient that maybe was unrelated to the patient's main complaint, he would use it as a teaching point."

In one instance of patient care conversation at the bedside, an attending asked of her team "Do you know the scratch test? You can't leave the service without learning this maneuver." And when an eager learner lit up and said he knew how, the attending asked him to demonstrate on the patient after obtaining permission. "Please show us how." The attending watched with careful intent as did the rest of the team. After a moment, she chimed in and laid hands on the patient also stating, "I do it with a slightly different technique. Take a look." The appreciation was palpable afterward with the medical student on the team saying with no small amount of awe, "That's pretty cool."

We saw an attending in the process of examining a patient hospitalized for a different reason point out a series of yellow globules on a patient's chest, indicative of damage from sun exposure. When his team of learners was in the room of a patient with cyclic vomiting, that same attending invited them to examine the patient's teeth, even though the patient had not mentioned any dental problems. The attending knew they would find damage caused by regurgitation of stomach acid.

One of the hallmarks of the 18 attendings is the thoroughness with which they approach both patient care and their teaching responsibilities. A former learner recalled an extreme example of that dedication, a visit he made to a patient with his attending and nine other learners. The attending wanted the learners to listen to the patient's lungs as the patient said "Eeee."[6] His attending, the former learner said, was not one of those teachers who would do the test himself and say, "Oh, he's got egophony," and then tell the team members to come back and do the test on their own time, knowing that most of them would never make it back. This attending insisted that every member of the team, one after the other, put their stethoscopes to the patient's chest while the patient pronounced the "Eeee." "We stood there," the former learner said, "the whole team. It must have taken 20 minutes, you know, with the attending apologizing to the patient, being nice to the patient. It was kind of funny, and the patient was laughing by the end of it, but that was how he did it. He was very thorough."

Inevitably, with a group of people conducting a physical examination on the same patient, differences of opinion will arise. One of the 18 attendings told us how he handles that situation. "We're going to listen together, look together, feel together," he said, "and I discipline myself to ask the learner, 'What did you hear, what did you see, what did you feel?' before I say anything."

The attending gave an example of a resident who said, "I think that's a diastolic murmur." The attending was confident it was systolic, but he did not say so directly so as not to undermine the resident's confidence. Instead, he told her, "Maybe I got this wrong. Let me listen again." And he taught her the technique of listening and, at the same time, matching the murmur to the pulse. "Then I didn't have to do anything more," the attending said. "She was able to say, 'Oh, yeah, that's systolic.'" He described how an exam disagreement with a learner should proceed.

> If we're in agreement, that's great; if we're not in agreement, then I re-examine with the learner. If we're still not in agreement, I say, "Let's listen right here and listen very specifically for this or let's feel right here and what do you feel now?" If that doesn't work, then we're going to have to come back in the afternoon.

Preparing for Possibilities

On patient rounds, one of the 18 attendings told us, she follows an "on-the-fly" teaching style. "It depends on what comes up on a day-to-day basis," she said. "So like, when we first saw the woman with the traumatic brain injury, we walk in and she's got the sand bed and so we talk about mattress choices, about turning schedules, about sacral decubitus ulcers. If somebody has a catheter, it's let's (a) take it out and (b) talk about catheter-related UTIs." This ensures that teaching is always in the context of the individual patient.

Spontaneity, however, is just one aspect of our attendings' conduct of patient rounds. Indeed, purely spontaneous teaching was a rarity. Nearly all attendings had prepared for rounds in advance by reading charts, reviewing clinical details, considering points in which learners might get stuck in their thought processes, and reviewing pertinent literature to share with the team. All before rounds even took place (see Figure 6.1). Based on what they had learned and their

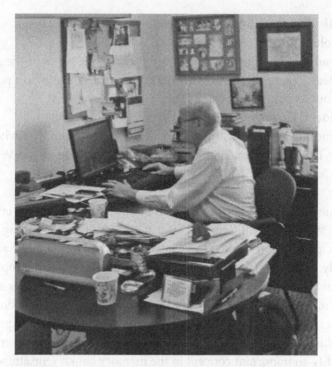

Figure 6.1 Attending reading over a patient's record.

knowledge of their team of learners, the attendings conjured up relevant teaching points and clarifications in advance. So, in most cases, rounds manifested as a combination of attendings' impromptu insights (inspired by the events of the particular patient encounter) and their calculated lessons and teaching points.

"I get here early to look over all my patients," one of the attendings told us, "so I already know what the team should be telling me, and I already know what I want to teach them." He always has one simple teaching point to make and one higher level point. For instance, he said, "A patient is on subcutaneous heparin, scheduled for surgery the next morning, and I will ask, 'How soon do we need to stop the heparin?' After that, I'll move on to something more involved, I'll say, 'Now, let's go to subcutaneous Lovenox.'"

The "on-the-fly" attending presided over the following exchange after a medical student presented on a patient:

Medical Student: So we should continue with LR [lactated Ringer's solution]?

Attending: I'm going to make my LR face. [She turns to the resident.] There's a paper on my desk, and we're going to do a point-counterpoint about using LR.

Resident: I'm not defending it.

Attending: But you will be. [She addresses the team as a whole.] When we come out of the patient's room, someone tell me: What's a fever?

The exchange initially appears to be simply an example of effortless, spontaneous instruction. But it turns out the attending had anticipated the reference to lactated Ringer's solution and had already carefully planned a more detailed discussion of the topic to occur later, with accompanying evidence from the medical literature.

The attendings especially like to scope out learner confusion or errors ahead of time so they can take full advantage of these prized teaching moments—nothing like a stuck point, yours or others', to solidify an important concept in the memory banks. One attending told us he can anticipate where his learners will be "stuck" with about 70% of patients. For 10% of patients, he added, "I will be stuck myself at the start and have to try to figure out what's going on." Another attending added: "I am always ahead of the house staff, though I may not let them know it. I feel most comfortable that way, anticipating and then giving them the space to catch up." That kind of preparation was nearly universal.

An attending gave us the backstory for a teaching moment we had witnessed earlier. He had seen the patient and gone over the notes a learner had prepared, and he was confident that the learner had missed a significant symptom. "So, I kind of went into that room," he said, "knowing we may find something here that's different from what I've read going in." Later, in the hallway, the learner and the other members of the team benefitted from the attending's insight. "It helps them pay attention at the bedside," he said. "Much of what I've learned about interviewing patients I've learned from watching other people do it." Indeed, there is value in observing a role model conduct clinical examination skills, a concept we return to in a future chapter.

Tailored Teaching and Bidirectional Feedback

The 18 attendings work hard at tailoring their teaching to the different needs of the individual team members, whether at the bedside, during table rounds, or during teaching sessions. It is no simple feat. Medical students, interns, and residents are, by definition, at different stages of their medical education and experience, and even within the same level of learner, individuals have unique learning styles, backgrounds, specialty interests, and sophistication.

A former learner said his attending taught "to every level of learner," offering this example of graduated complexity: "She would start out talking about the lab abnormalities when a liver is not functioning well, which is practical information no matter what specialty a learner is interested in. But then she would get into our patient's cirrhosis and the details of how to manage it."

Given the different educational levels in a team, though, there will always be moments when one or another learner doesn't understand some aspect of an explanation. Because they are superb diagnosticians and have carefully honed attention to their patients and their learners, the 18 attendings keep a keen eye out for what one of them called "that blank look." She expounded on this and highlighted an important and often-discussed concept of making explicit one's own clinical thought evolution and reasoning through words: "I try to talk through processes out loud as much as possible, because I think sometimes we jump from Point A to Point C and we skip Point B in the middle." That jump can easily cause the blank look to appear on learners' faces. When that happens, the attending said, "I just let it go, and go back to the learner later. And I go through the material again with him until he says, 'Okay, now it makes sense.' We can't leave them with these big open gaps in the knowledge they need to take to the next patient." If and when teaching attendings notice learners' blank looks, they make it a point to rephrase or reframe the question and approach it from a different angle until the learner becomes unstuck.

Our attendings provide learners with a maximum of individual attention through one-on-one meetings. At these sessions, the learners are invited to share any questions or uncertainties about the clinical concepts being discussed. Indeed, at the beginning of a rotation, some attendings urge learners to keep a written list of items they would like to learn more about and concepts they are uncertain about for later discussion with the attendings.

In addition to clarifying concepts and giving learners feedback, attendings use the one-on-one meetings to solicit feedback from their learners for ideas to improve their own teaching. "I tell them I'm trying to get better every day, too," an attending said, "and so, what can I do differently that would help you learn better? I had a senior resident who told me I was being too hard on the interns. That's fine! I found ways to build them up."

Another attending offers an unusual individual service for the medical students on his team. He has them print paper copies of the notes they enter into the electronic medical record. "I'll get out a red pen, just for fun," the attending said, "and I'll put on this frowny face, and I'll mark up their H&Ps [history and physicals] and tell them to go back over them." It takes 10 minutes for each document review, a strain on the attending's schedule, but he knows how valuable it is for learners. "If someone had done that for me," he said, "I would have been in a lot better shape. I had no idea how to do a note [as a student]."

The attendings put substantial effort into providing high-yield, detailed feedback about the interactions and events unfolding within the patient's room. To provide specific, measurable, and actionable feedback, attendings may capture these detailed events by taking careful notes. In a particular noteworthy example, one teaching attending provides daily feedback, delivered via email, to the team's senior resident after bedside rounds have concluded. The attending characterizes this feedback:

> You asked this question, and it was an awkward moment. If you had just asked this person first, it could have been a much smoother interaction.

We were in that room too long. We boxed out the nurse when we were at bedside.

And here's the senior resident's characterization of the attending's feedback:

> Every afternoon after rounds, I get an email from him with a PDF of his notes from morning rounds. It really is step-by-step, what I said, what I should have said, what my body position was, whether something was good or what I could improve upon. It's extremely helpful because a lot of my actions on rounds are subconscious, and I don't realize that I am doing it.

Distinctive Teaching Styles

On patient rounds or during table rounds, the 18 attendings have their own distinctive styles of teaching (see Figure 6.2). Some

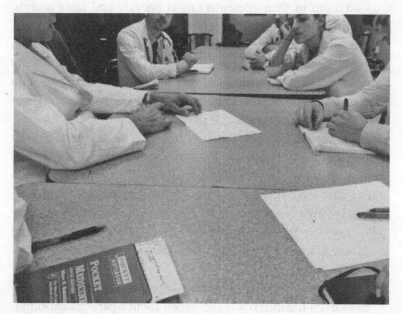

Figure 6.2 Table rounds with the team.

will deliver a five-minute discourse in the hallway after seeing a patient, typically because the topic is so spot-on to the patient's main concern and the context is so fresh. Others are more inclined to save their teaching sessions for table rounds. But all of the attendings have at their mental beck and call dozens of so-called *teaching scripts* (short lectures that deal with particular diseases or findings such as an approach to hyponatremia). Their mastery of the scripts gives attendings the ability to vary the length of their presentation depending on the venue: shorter at the bedside, longer during table rounds or dedicated teaching sessions.

According to their learners, current and former, the attendings deliver "high-yield" lectures. "I think he understands really well . . . where we are coming from," a current learner said of his attending. "He can teach us a whole humongous topic in 15 minutes, and we all, in the end, probably have a better understanding than if we sat down with a textbook for three hours. That's happened multiple times this week already."

In addition to their presentations at bedside and table rounds, some of the attendings will, once or twice a week, gather the medical students on their teams for a brief lecture, usually no more than 10 minutes, geared to their learning level (see Figure 6.3). "That's one thing I took away from him," a former student said. "Now I do these clinical pearl talks too, like from aortic stenosis to central line-associated bloodstream infections."

The 18 attendings look for ways to pique the learners' interest in their lectures, beyond the learners' interest in expanding their knowledge about their chosen profession. They will often use a joke or a topical reference to make it more relevant and cement the contents of their discussion into the learners' memories.

We saw the following table rounds exchange after an intern presented on a patient who had an unexplained stroke:

Intern: I'm thinking DVT [deep vein thrombosis] and getting an ultrasound. [The intern was concerned about a paradoxical embolism due to a heart defect.]

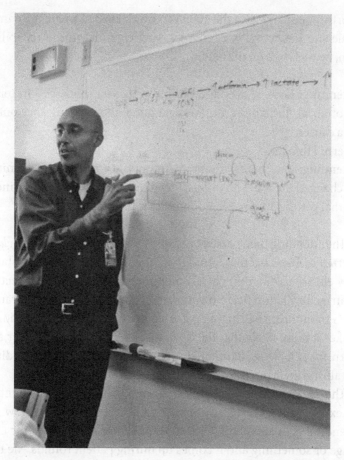

Figure 6.3 Attending conducting a short teaching session after rounds.

Attending: I think that's perfect. In terms of diagnosing, let's say it is negative.

Intern: I'm not entirely certain. . . .

Attending: It's controversial. The opinions wax and wane. Are you football fans?

At that point, the attending pulled several copies of an article from his pocket and handed them around. It was about the New England Patriots defensive star, Tedy Bruschi, who suffered a mild stroke shortly after playing in the 2005 Pro Bowl. He had a patent foramen ovale and was partially paralyzed. After eight months of rehabilitation, he was back on the field.

Attending: Look it over and tell me what you think. . . . In terms of atrial fibrillation, do you feel good about ruling that out as a cause?
Intern: I think so.
Attending: So, here's another [important] article. It definitely changed the way I do things. I read this article and was convinced that getting 30-day event monitors is the right thing to do.

The attending then passed out a 2014 article from the *New England Journal of Medicine* that found that 30 days of noninvasive ambulatory electrocardiogram (ECG) monitoring improved the detection of atrial fibrillation fivefold compared with standard short-duration ECG monitoring.[7] Bringing paper copies of articles to table rounds makes it more likely that the team will look through the paper and learn from it while simultaneously demonstrating how attendings are always incorporating research into their practice.

The 18 attendings have different ways of providing or pointing to extra reading material. A current learner described how his attending goes about it. "If we've been talking about antibiotic coverage or something and it comes up during patient rounds," he told us, "she'll hop onto the computer right there and pull things up and show them to you. Or she'll forward us papers, like right after rounds. If you like evidence-based medicine, it's nice to see that." Nor does the attending forget that she sent the material. "The next time the same problem appears," the learner said, "she'll be like: 'So did you read those guidelines we talked about?'"

Other teaching attendings recognize that younger learners are tending to rely on more bite-sized methods of learning. This may be captured best by one attending who quipped, "Communication with [younger learners] is different. I mean, email is now a carrier pigeon. You have to text or you tweet or whatever." Some harness technologies like smartphones to show representative images of visual diagnoses or auditory physical examination findings (see Figure 6.4). Others recognize the preference of some learners for asynchronous communication and learning, using group texting to discuss clinical questions that arise on rounds. Still others take advantage of different learning styles and vehicles, pointing learners toward podcasts, videos, and Twitter feeds (so-called *tweetorials*, longer threads of tweets that illustrate a clinical concept or answer a question, are especially popular within medical education communities).

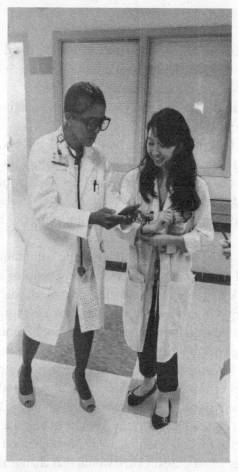

Figure 6.4 Attending using a smartphone to show an image on rounds.

The 18 attendings are alert to topics that may go uncovered. For example, some topics reviewed by attendings include lectures on billing and coding, communication skills, different types of healthcare systems, patient safety, and medical ethics. Another of our attendings reviewed with her team a list of nursing homes she has found to be reliable. "I don't think any residency does a really good job of preparing residents for the transition to being a faculty member," she said.

We close this chapter with a potpourri of teaching ideas and techniques our attendings employ.

- Memorized teaching scripts are a staple of a medical educator's toolkit, developed and refined over years. Several of the attendings share their scripts with the learners. As one said, "They can do whatever they want with them, ignore it, modify it, adapt it to your needs."
- "I have long believed that learners like the people who are teaching them to be *smart*," one of our attendings said. "So, for the first few sessions in a month, I try to show overwhelming knowledge of medicine to dazzle a little." It also, he added, suggests to learners that these "dazzling things are a part of their future."
- When a team orders a test, there is an assumption that the result will be positive. "I always say," an attending told us, "presume it is negative so that whatever happens, you can go to the next step. Otherwise, if it doesn't show anything, you are all going to be sitting there in the same spot." Some refer to this teaching technique as "anticipatory medicine," and it helps the team to feel prepared for as many patient outcomes as possible. This was echoed by several. For instance, one attending was quoted as saying "I want you to think about what you'll do if the scan comes back negative." Another posed a hypothetical scenario to make a teaching point: "Let's pretend her diarrhea increases when she eats. How would that change things in your minds?"

- A popular device among attending physicians in general—and for our 18 as well—is the *mnemonic*, a word whose letters typically represent a medical grouping, such as the names of the bones in the hand or the symptoms of a disease.[8] For example, a classic mnemonic for recalling the indications for acute hemodialysis is "A-E-I-O-U," which stands for Acidosis, Electrolyte disturbance, Intoxication, volume Overload, and Uremia.

- One attending carries a whiteboard about with him, using it to take notes—lab values during rounds, for example—or to sketch parts of the body during a table rounds lecture or a bedside talk. A current learner compared his attending's sketches to looking at a PowerPoint presentation on a screen: "It's complete night and day in terms of being able to follow along and pay attention and be invested in what's being taught." (Other attendings use index cards to the same effect.)

- Another attending plays a game called "Around the World." If he has a question that has multiple correct answers, he calls on each team member to give one answer, starting with the medical students. Saying "I don't know" is allowed and met with nonjudgment. "I have to play, too," the attending said, "and if it gets to me a second time, it's really hard." One team played this game by reviewing various causes of cancer-induced high calcium levels in the blood.

A current learner of one of the 18 attendings summed up much of what we have written about in this chapter: "The most important thing wasn't getting out on time or showing you knew more than anybody else. The most important thing was to be with the patient at the bedside, caring for them and their families. That's why you were there and that's why you were a doctor."

In the following chapter, we consider another important aspect of clinical education: the attending's thought process and how it is applied and shared with their learners. Among other matters, we explore the Socratic method of questioning and the value of second thoughts.

Main Points

1. The attendings make bedside teaching (or the teaching that occurs just outside of a patient's room) a mainstay of their approach. They feel that the best way to learn is from patients themselves. They combine their physical examination and questioning of the patient with the presentation of relevant teaching points.

2. Attendings teach that information learned from a current patient should be applied to the next relevant patient. In this way, what is taught builds on itself, creating a solid foundation of knowledge.

3. Attendings not only teach to the team but are also alert to any need to provide individual instruction. They recognize that team members have different learning capacities and seek to prevent knowledge gaps from developing in every level of learner.

Further Reading

Peters M, Ten Cate O. Bedside teaching in medical education: A literature review. Perspect Med Educ 2014;3:76–88.

   In this article, the authors conducted a literature review on the use of bedside teaching in medical education. Although bedside teaching was once the primary modality for teaching clinical skills, its use has declined in recent years. Thus, the authors sought to determine bedside teaching's role and strengths in teaching clinical skills and understand why its use has declined. The authors found that trainees and patients alike seem to value bedside teaching. But, because of shortened patient admissions and an increased reliance on technology to determine diagnosis, bedside teaching is on the decline.

Irby DM. Three exemplary models of case-based teaching. Acad Med 1994;69:947–53.

   In this article, Irby describes three distinctive ways of organizing teaching rounds: (1) case-bedside teaching, (2) case-lecture teaching, and (3) case-iterative teaching. These three models of teaching share five common characteristics, including anchoring instruction in cases, actively involving learners in the process of teaching, modeling professional thinking and action, providing direction and feedback, and creating collaborative learning environments. Incorporating these five characteristics into the teaching process will facilitate the learning process.

McMahon GT, Marina O, Kritek PA, Katz JT. Effect of a physical examination teaching program on the behavior of medical residents. J Gen Intern Med 2005;20:710–4.

Although the physical examination is a critical component in determining a diagnosis, its use as a diagnostic aid has declined. Thus, this study conducted a series of educational workshops for medical residents to determine whether such a program could increase the use of the physical examination among medical residents. After the program, there was a marked improvement in performance of the physical exam on rounds, and residents reported that their exam skills improved, as did their ability to teach these skills.

Ramani S. Twelve tips for excellent physical examination teaching. Med Teach 2008;30:851–6.

In this article, Ramani describes the key challenges in teaching the physical examination and offers 12 practical strategies that institutions and educators can use to promote high-quality physical exam teaching. The author describes the importance of the physical exam as it relates to patient–physician interactions and its role in the clinical diagnosis process.

7

How to Think About Thinking

Thought is the blossom; language the bud; action the fruit behind it.

—Ralph Waldo Emerson

One current learner told us that he was mystified. "I don't know how she does it," he said of his attending physician, "but she teaches you without *teaching* you."

By the time many learners start their clinical rotations, they have spent years with teachers who provided them, through discussion, readings, and resources, with all the required information. The students were expected to listen, read, and memorize for the final exam.

Our 18 outstanding attending physicians have a very different teaching style. Their strategy was active rather than passive, collaborative rather than authoritarian. "I approach it as more of a dialogue than a teaching," one of them told us. Another added: "I stimulate them to think and work through the problems as opposed to me just telling them the answer."

In the team approach to clinical education, senior members, including the attendings, oversee the learning experiences of junior members all while monitoring patients' care and learners' progress. They also look for potential teaching moments to lead learners beyond simple recall questions about a patient's ailments toward higher level questions. The goal: to help learners develop both the analytic and the intuitive components of clinical reasoning, the sine qua non of medical practice.

Teaching Inpatient Medicine. Second Edition. Nathan Houchens, Molly Harrod, and Sanjay Saint, Oxford University Press. © Nathan Houchens, Molly Harrod, and Sanjay Saint 2023.
DOI: 10.1093/oso/9780197639023.003.0007

In this chapter, we describe how the 18 attendings go about that task—in essence, how they think about thinking and teach without teaching. We will explore the fundamental role questions play in fostering clinical reasoning as well as the ways in which attendings develop and ask their questions, share their own thought processes, and implant a desire for lifelong learning in their team members.

Clinical Reasoning

In this context, clinical reasoning is the set of skills used by physicians to correctly diagnose patients' conditions and develop appropriate treatments. It has two main components. The first is the ability to mentally stockpile and integrate information gathered in the process of treating vast numbers of patients and reading vast quantities of research studies and clinical resources. Physicians thereby learn to recognize patterns of clinical data, and that sometimes makes it possible for them to make almost reflexive and automatic diagnoses. This process, known as a type of cognitive heuristic or mental shortcut, is rapid, intuitive, and nonanalytical.

The second major facet of physicians' clinical reasoning is more methodical and analytical. Physicians painstakingly examine and weigh all the evidence, including the clinical history and physical examination, to generate probabilities that then inform next steps. Hypotheses are developed, tested, and retested on the path toward a differential diagnosis and a management plan.

Although quite different, the two components of clinical reasoning are complementary. In most cases, both analytical and nonanalytical elements are intertwined and play a role in eventual decisions. Care must be exercised with heuristics, however. Studies have shown that an overreliance on the intuitive leap to diagnosis can lead to error.[1]

Clinical education has always tilted toward the analytical component of clinical reasoning. Learners spend their days examining patients and weighing differential diagnoses in terms of their probability. But many attendings, including our 18, also acknowledge in their teaching the intuitive aspects of clinical care.[2]

"Moving from intern to resident," one attending told us about patterns of recognition, "gives you the ability to determine when a patient is sick or not. You have seen the spectrum of sick to not sick; you have processed thousands of pieces of information. Then, wow, something's different about a patient. And when you decide [to call a rapid response team], it's a visceral, gut feeling, and you have to trust yourself."

Another of our attendings said that he teaches using the questions he asks himself when considering a patient—questions that may cast doubt on accepted recommendations. "Where the questions come from, I don't know," he continued. "Sometimes it's just a vision: Well, this is odd. Why is this?" Effective questioning is a most useful tool in the attending physician's armamentarium.

Teaching Arises from Questions

Questions posed, either to the self or to team members, form the foundation of teaching by revealing learning opportunities. Purposeful and carefully crafted questions are essential to explore the level of learners' comprehension and to guide their thought processes. "If a question comes to me [from the attending]," a current learner told us, "there's a reason it comes to me. I never feel that the attending is trying to put me in a place where I won't know the answer to the question. I think he's trying to assay the frontier of my knowledge. And I think the question is based on patients that I've seen recently, so it's not completely out of the blue."

The attendings' questions serve another purpose: they inspire the *modest* degree of anxiety that makes learners more receptive to learning. Note the emphasis on "modest." As indicated in earlier chapters, our attendings go to great lengths to create a supportive, noncompetitive team environment for learners that minimizes insecurity and anxiety.[3] Yet our attendings also realize that complacency undermines learning and breeds poor patient care. Indeed, one way of thinking about how some attendings approach learning is to consider the relationship between learning and stress as depicted

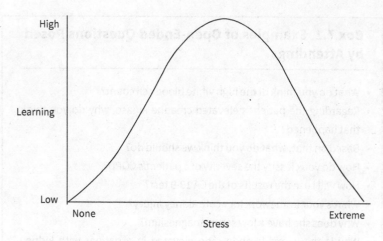

Figure 7.1 Learning–stress curve.

in Figure 7.1. This inverted U-shaped relationship indicates that learning is compromised with too little or too much anxiety. Finding that right balance of stress and support—that optimizes motivation and avoids the overwhelmed feeling—is what attendings seek.

Most of the attendings' queries ask learners what conclusions they have reached about their patients with respect to diagnosis and treatment. At times, a single exchange of fact-based recall inquiries will suffice: "What dose would you give?" "When would you restart the medication?" More often, however, attendings will inquire about a learner's thought process using open-ended questions (see Box 7.1).

The attending takes a learner through a series of questions that carry the learner from interpretation of data to determination of a diagnosis to settling on a treatment plan to decisions of what to do if the unexpected occurs or the plan falters. All along the way, the attending is probing to determine the level of the learner's understanding of the patient's condition.

In their probing, the 18 attendings frequently employ hypothetical questions centered on what-if scenarios to spur learners to think outside their comfort zones and prepare for all possible outcomes. This is referred to by some as "anticipatory medicine." Diagnostic tests are often ordered on the expectation that they

---

Box 7.1 Examples of Open-Ended Questions Posed by Attendings

- What do you think of the high white blood cell count?
- Regarding the patient's elevated creatine kinase, why do you think that happened?
- Based on that, what do you think we should do?
- How do you classify the severity of a patient's COPD?
- How will I use the results of the CA 19-9 test?
- What's your framework for acute kidney injury?
- Why does she have a low serum magnesium?
- Why is the kappa-lambda ratio elevated in a patient with kidney disease?
- If he doesn't improve after this dose, how would you like to proceed?

---

will return positive, thus supporting the validity of a diagnosis. Medications and other treatments are often ordered presuming that they will have the desired effect of alleviating suffering or ameliorating the condition. The what-if questions require learners to consider the impact of a negative result or lack of treatment response on their mental picture of the patient. As one former learner put it, "[The attending] uses a Wayne Gretzky quote about skating 'to where the puck is going to be' versus skating to where the puck is. A lot of the things he teaches us are about predicting changes and predicting things. So, on rounds, he is always referring to, this might happen, we are going to prepare for this. Things like that."

Along with hypotheticals, the attendings' questions often raise alternatives to the existing diagnosis or treatment plan, another challenge that forces learners to come up with a different way of thinking about the patient. Hypotheticals and alternatives place learners into circumstances that they are likely to face in the future as full-fledged practicing physicians. The questions serve as a vehicle to simulate authentic situations in which their conclusions are challenged and they are forced to reconsider on their feet, in the middle of the action, with little or no time for preparation. These scenarios can also serve as jumping-off points for discussion that moves learners beyond the individual patient toward future patients, higher level topics, and more robust understanding.

A simple but powerful technique our attendings employed frequently was to ask learners to verbalize their thought processes. "How do you approach a patient with fever of unknown origin?" "What makes you think that?" Thinking aloud and providing rationale for decisions makes space for reflection. And when the attending also verbalizes their own thinking, a community of practice and shared understanding takes shape. One learner summarized this as follows: "I had to actually think about why I wanted to do things, and then I was allowed to do them. I remember specifically wanting to do a cosyntropin stim test on a patient, and he told me I had to explain why I needed to do that before we proceeded with ordering the test and actually doing it myself. So, in that regard, he was very invested in me trying to learn."

Learners' critical thinking is not, the 18 attendings insist, supposed to stop once a better plan is conceived. Learners are urged to constantly rethink their conclusions, reassess their priorities, and debrief after challenging situations. Indeed, consistently questioning conclusions, from any member of the team, is expected and viewed by our attendings as a positive behavior rather than a lack of confidence. We often heard the attendings say, "Looking back to last night, what else could we have done?" or something similar. They also often invite their learners to ask them questions and engage in healthy and generative debate. "When we can successfully stimulate our students to ask their own questions," says a professor in a study of college teaching, "we are laying the foundation for learning."[4] As a former learner stated when asked about their attending: "You can very easily disagree with him and challenge him, say that, no, that's not the case . . . you can say whatever you think or you can say that you disagree." The following prompts, put forth back-to-back by an attending to her team, illustrate the concept:

Attending: So, the question is what happened last night with our patient that developed hypothermia? What are your thoughts?

Attending: Let's say you get a cross-cover call and it's a patient with hypothermia. What are you going to do?

Another type of question our attendings sometimes use might be called a non-question or check-in question. It is asked not so much to elicit information as to inspire second thoughts. Two current learners recalled an example:

First learner: A lot of times, when he says, "Oh, did that guy get a CT scan?" Whether I do or don't recall ordering the test, it makes me second-guess myself. I double-check my work. It makes you go back and review and really know your patients better.

Second learner: When he asked about the CT scan, I think he knew that it wasn't done, you know, but it made them question, "Does the patient need a CT scan?"

First learner: That may be just his way of asking us, you know, did we really complete our workup? His nice way of saying, "Did we do everything we should have for this patient?"

Sometimes no question is required at all. Attendings may inspire learners to determine for themselves which points of information about a patient are important, as in the following exchange:

Medical student: [To attending] Do you want me to share any other laboratory results?

Attending: Not unless *you* think they're important.

The Socratic Philosophy

The most challenging (and perhaps rewarding) type of questioning our attending physicians pursue is rooted in the so-called *Socratic method*, credited to the ancient Greek philosopher, Socrates. Legend has it that Socrates thought it no accident that his mother was a mid-wife because his teaching technique helped students give birth to new ideas.[5]

The Socratic technique calls for the teacher to ask a student a series of linked questions, each question built on the previous answer, thus leading to the self-discovery of a truth that had existed, unrecognized, in the student's brain. Teaching, as it were, without teaching.

Socratic questions put forth by the 18 attendings are not intended to determine learners' knowledge levels. The attendings already know that part of their responsibility is recognizing individual learners' areas of strength and weakness to help them improve. In other words, attendings routinely diagnose their learners as well as their patients. So, as the questions move in a logical sequence from one concept to the next, learners can respond to the attendings' questions and make mental connections all the way to their conclusion. The goal is to guide the learners to a new, richer level of understanding. A current learner told us of his experience with the Socratic method.

[Attendings] gauge where your knowledge is and then sort of put themselves in your brain and lead you down the path. They don't start the questions at a higher level, such that you would be like, "I just don't know that." Instead, they start slowly, and they sort of leave a trail of breadcrumbs for you to follow so that you're making connections all along the way. And you come out of that conversation feeling good, because you came to the right place in the end.

Here is an illustrative example of the Socratic method in practice, outlined by one attending physician's probing questions to her team regarding a patient with fluid around the heart (pericardial effusion):

- What thoughts do you have about this patient's pericardial effusion?
- What is the most dangerous form of pericardial effusion?
- What physical examination findings point you in the direction of pericardial tamponade?

- What do you remember about that eponymous Beck's triad?
- What is your approach to measuring pulsus paradoxus?
- What are your thoughts on the hemodynamic changes that can lead a patient to get worse?

On the very next patient seen by this attending, another pristine example of open-ended, Socratic questioning emerged.

Attending: Tell me about the acid–base issues with salicylate toxicity.

Medical student: It causes acidosis.

Attending: Great! Is that a metabolic or respiratory acidosis?

[A short while later]

Attending: Is metabolic acidosis the only acid–base disorder in salicylate poisoning?

Medical student: Well, actually you have to be sure you're looking at the pH and bicarbonate to ensure it's not a mixed picture. In this case, he also has respiratory alkalosis.

Attending: Nice work, you got it! So . . . when I read about this next piece, it was a real lightbulb moment for me. Ingesting other substances that depress the respiratory rate can cloud the acid–base picture. . . . Now, let's tie this concept back to our previous conversation about the indications for acute hemodialysis. . . .

Frameworks and Conceptual Learning

The attendings' emphasis is always on learners' thought processes, rather than on the details of their work. There is no conceivable way learners can memorize all the facts involved in practicing medicine. What they can and must master are the methods: the ways of thinking that enable physicians to cope with their everyday challenges. This often takes the form of frameworks, schemas, and conceptual models, a method popularized by some online references.[6]

"Rather than feeding us factual information," a current learner said of his attending, "he teaches us the heuristics of medicine—how to approach a problem—so that we have a framework for going about it." That included learning to synthesize the key aspects of a patient's condition, identifying the "major points, the big decisions." One attending made this explicit when describing her approach to pulmonary function test interpretation: "I don't memorize the diagnostic criteria. I have to decide what to use my brain space for. I just want to introduce you to the concept; I don't want you to memorize it."

There will always be patients who present new and different problems. There will always be new research results, medications, and treatments to integrate into physicians' knowledge base and practice. To cope with such challenges, physicians will need to maintain that ability to use frameworks, to think about thinking like they practiced during clinical rounds. A current learner recalled hearing a speech by one of our 18 attendings.

> He talked about how you have to constantly be improving . . . constantly be actively learning. He talked about just how he is kind of obsessed with reading journals. I found it very inspiring. He is so dedicated to improving himself, and he so thoroughly enjoys what he does. I think that's how you get to be a doctor of his caliber.

On the topic of reviewing medical journals and literature, our attendings go beyond assigning readings. Instead, they frequently demonstrate just how they critically analyze journal articles rather than simply accepting their results. In point of fact, they encouraged learners to ask their own questions of the article and its authors. This technique spurs learners to deeper comprehension and recall than does simple passive absorption of the article's main points. And when clinical questions arise on rounds that are not well described in the scholarly literature? Our attendings would sometimes pose questions like "How would you fill that knowledge gap?" Questions like these challenge learners to craft their own hypothetical research study that would help to answer the question.

In addition to their teaching, attending physicians also serve—consciously or unconsciously—as role models for their learners. In the following chapter, we look at some of the ways in which our 18 attendings fulfil that responsibility. Topics include the uncertainty principle and the hidden curriculum, patience and perseverance, and mortality and joy.

Main Points

1. Attendings view the use of higher-order, open-ended questions as effective teaching vehicles.
2. Questions serve multiple purposes, including guiding learners through their thinking processes, building on knowledge through the use of hypothetical questions, and using the Socratic method to foster critical thinking.
3. Instilling the ability to think critically about one's own decision-making process is the attendings' ultimate goal for their learners.

Further Reading

Tversky A, Kahneman D. Judgment under uncertainty: Heuristics and biases. Science 1974;185:1124–31.

In this classic 1974 article, Tversky and Kahneman address human biases by examining the ways in which people generally make judgments in uncertain conditions. Heuristics that allow us to make such decisions are often necessary, but they can also create severe, systematic errors in decision-making. The authors examine three common heuristics and delineate the associated biases these can lead to: representativeness, availability, and adjustment and anchoring. Broadly, *representativeness* leads to several biases based on stereotyping and inappropriate extrapolation. *Availability* can lead to several biases, such as instance retrievability, imaginability, or illusory correlation. Finally, *adjustment and anchoring* combine to create less flexible thought processes. Anchoring particularly biases the resulting calculation toward the chosen starting point, leading to insufficient adjustment. Similarly, anchoring can lead to biased subjective probability distributions. In sum, the authors of this seminal article provide clear and convincing evidence of the ways in which our tendency to use heuristics can bias our thinking and thus impact patient health.

Pichan C, Dhaliwal G, Cusick A, Saint S, Houchens N. Inadequate support. N Engl J Med 2021;385:938–44.

In this clinical problem-solving piece from the *New England Journal of Medicine*, readers are presented a complex case with an unexpected conclusion. A 71-year-old man presented to the emergency room with a constellation of bleeding-related symptoms. After working through the differential diagnosis and keeping an open mind, the physicians in this case were able to track the cause of the patient's health condition back to a lack of vitamin C: scurvy. This condition—uncommon in the United States because of the ready availability of fruits and vegetables—may have been ignored or dismissed without keeping an open mind about potential causes and taking a thorough history from the patient.

Singh H, Connor DM, Dhaliwal G. Five strategies for clinicians to advance diagnostic excellence. BMJ 2022;376:e068044.

The mark of many an excellent physician is diagnostic excellence, a mastery that can only be obtained from intentional and sustained effort. According to US and international health authorities, measuring and reducing diagnostic error is a key patient safety priority. Diagnosis is a process influenced by many factors (from systems to social) that can enhance or reduce diagnostic accuracy. The authors state that clinicians can leverage diagnostic performance feedback as a part of their daily work. A key area in which clinicians can take steps to mitigate biases is in relation to race, ethnicity, gender, or other identities. These types of biases may conflict with their values and thus can impair diagnostic accuracy. Clinicians can add expertise from other health professionals, patients, and families to reimagine every aspect of the diagnostic process. This article presents five strategies to improve a clinician's diagnostic excellence: (1) seek feedback on diagnostic decisions, (2) regularly challenge one's diagnostic acumen by testing diagnostic skill in challenges, (3) consider one's biases to avoid incorrect diagnostic conclusions, (4) make diagnosis a team sport by including as many voices from healthcare professionals as practicable, and (5) foster critical thinking by maintaining a skeptical attitude toward the diagnostic question, always seeking data to support or refute conclusions. Including examples and resources to maintain and improve diagnostic skill, this paper provides an excellent starting point when one wishes to improve their diagnostic acumen.

Detsky AS. Learning the art and science of diagnosis. JAMA 2022;327:1759–60.

Diagnosis is not simply a skill rooted in science and evidence, this author explains; it is also an art because the lines of decision can be very gray at times. All diagnoses begin by gathering data, which today come in multiple forms, from imaging studies, electronic medical records, and patient exams. The key for the physician is determining which of the many findings are useful in determining a diagnosis. This is an iterative process, with physicians using Bayesian thinking to compare relevant data points to known disease profiles while also potentially unveiling new information that may help whittle down the list of possible diagnoses. A list of disease signs or symptoms may not be enough, though, since diseases can present in multiple forms. Next comes determining the method of communication, which can be synchronous (direct person-to-person communication) or asynchronous (e.g., email or note in the electronic medical record). One can often determine the method needed by urgency or the need to have a nuanced interpretation of certain results by consultants. While technology has and will continue to offer partial or novel solutions, diagnosis must be made by the physician.

8

Role Models

> *Being a role model is equal parts being who you actually are and what people hope you will be.*
>
> —Meryl Streep

To one extent or another, for better or worse, attending physicians become their learners' role models. One survey found that 90% of a medical school's graduating class listed one or more physician role models identified during medical school, and that 63% of students had received career advice and counseling from these role models.[1] The 18 outstanding attendings we interviewed and observed take this aspect of their role very seriously. They understand that their behavior—as physicians, as instructors, as human beings—will likely be internalized and emulated by some of their learners. Given this important responsibility, they maintain a high bar and continually monitor their performance, striving to make sure that they are living up to their personal and professional standards.

Medical learners may embark on a certain career pathway because of an attending's influence. The former learner of one such attending explained how she had inspired him to go into hospital medicine. "I learned from her how to navigate people and systems in an inpatient environment, how to work well with lots of different people. She was my role model."

In the previous chapters, we discussed the 18 attendings' creation of supportive and team-based environments and their teaching techniques. In this chapter, we focus on some of the personal qualities, traits, and mindsets the attendings model and some of the

Teaching Inpatient Medicine. Second Edition. Nathan Houchens, Molly Harrod, and Sanjay Saint,
Oxford University Press. © Nathan Houchens, Molly Harrod, and Sanjay Saint 2023.
DOI: 10.1093/oso/9780197639023.003.0008

special challenges they confront in that endeavor. The ultimate goal in their role-modeling mission will be the focus of a future chapter: their treatment of and interactions with patients.

Devotion Through Diligence and Self-Discipline

Our attendings have high expectations for their team members—and for themselves. "I'm a perfectionist, and I have high standards for myself," one of the attendings said, "but I think it's really important to take each student as an individual and help them be the best *they* can be, not necessarily to my standards." Even those learners who have been directly told by an attending that they are not working as hard as they could know "deep inside," a former learner said, that the attending will protect them and work to "pull their good things [out of them]."

Once again, attendings were viewed as team members working alongside learners, rather than as authoritative bosses. That included diligence in all their work, both in front of the team and behind the scenes. "You know, he's working harder than anybody on the team," an attending's former learner said, "and that really sets the bar for how you expect yourself to work." Here's how another former learner described his attending's approach:

> He was as nice and calm as you could be with the students, the residents, and the patients, but in the background, he was doing as much hard work as anybody else, checking up on the patients, checking up on us, checking up on medications, reconciliations. While all that was happening, he had a very carefree approach during rounds, like, "this is easy, let's have fun." But in the background, that was never really the case. The informality makes everyone like him, makes everyone learn from him very well, and meanwhile he's very hands-on, doing things.

To maintain their myriad tasks as physician, teacher, and role model, the 18 attendings must be models of self-discipline. That can make for long days and nights. "My attending gets up at 4 o'clock every morning and reads the journals," a current learner told us in admiration and wonder. His colleague added: "When I think about him, discipline comes to mind."

A key element of the attendings' self-discipline is their routine monitoring of their own performance. They understand that reflection on successes and challenges can help them accomplish their goal of continuous improvement. In fact, as one study found, the more frequently check-ups on progress occur, the more likely success is achieved.[2]

Our attendings make it clear to their teams that physicians must never rest on their laurels but must always strive to be even better versions of themselves. "He is the most knowledgeable person," a learner said of his attending, "yet even he himself admits you're never perfect and you've just got to keep on learning." The attendings are constantly looking for ways to improve their skills, and their learners know it. One of the attendings told us about reviewing the literature to find articles that will "make me a better doctor and maybe a better teacher." Another spoke of his effort to live up to his own role models: "What inspired me was I had role models in my life that just [made me say] 'I want to be like that' and I'm still trying to 'be like that.'" Another echoed this method of learning from others, often trusted peers and individuals the attendings wish to emulate.

> My teaching now is better than it was five years ago, and I bet it will be better five years from now. You know, when I do something good, but someone does it even better, I love to hear about it. Because, you know, you are on a personal quest to do better and better, but your own creativity is limited, and someone else's creativity is limitless.

One attending talked about how to improve teaching competence through the iterative cycles of direct observation and thoughtful reflection. His team, he said, "should go watch other attendings teach and then reflect carefully about what they learned and how it could be used to improve their own teaching skills." In fact, he went on, that's what he and the other attendings have been doing: "All of us have gotten better, I think, over the years I've been here, and in part it's because we are watching each other."

Behind the attendings' commitment to self-improvement is their core belief in the value of the larger medical enterprise. They care about their legacy as part of that enterprise and work to ensure they pass along key principles to future generations of physicians. "My job is to tell you what I know and to make sure that, at the end, you know more than I do," one of the 18 attendings told us, "and to make sure that I have inspired you to do that to the people who come after you." That is how they present themselves to their teams. "You see his devotion to a cause he feels is his calling in life," a learner said of his attending, "and you can see yourself trying your best to emulate that."

The Hidden Curriculum

As teachers and role models, attendings should be conscious of another formidable force that can influence their learners—what one article describes as "the informal and hidden curricula that are ubiquitous in hospitals and medical schools."[3] The hidden curriculum consists of a set of values, beliefs, and behaviors that are seldom said aloud but are widely accepted and practiced within hospitals, for good or ill. In essence, it encompasses local culture and norms, and it represents another kind of role model for learners—a model that may foster inspiration and good, or that may perpetuate problematic ideas and undermine the efforts of well-meaning and responsible attending physicians.

In their treatment of patients, for example, the hospital's mores may emphasize efficiency over empathy, such that physicians may pay little attention to patients' emotional concerns. Provider empathy has been shown to have clear positive influences on patients' health, is key to achieving patient-centeredness in the hospital, and is a defined educational objective in US medical training.[4,5] Despite this, a systematic review of the literature showed that there is a decline in self-assessed empathy among learners as training progresses.

Several aspects of the hidden curriculum are cited as potential causes of this empathy drop. Mistreatment by superiors and medical student vulnerability, the reality of suffering and death, a shift in focus toward technology and objectivity, social support problems, and high workload are all common denominators.[4]

Additionally, hierarchies and groupings of team members may lead to a number of challenges: other non-physician members of the healthcare team may be treated less as partners and more as subordinates. Learners may be expected to be deferential, even subservient, to more senior members of the team.

During our interviews of the 18 attendings' team members and former learners, we often encountered veiled references to the hidden curriculum. They spoke of other physicians who had demeaned them in front of their peers or were "so intimidating you're afraid to talk or communicate with them." They expressed relief that their attending (one of the 18) "doesn't have this need to have the last say because of his position" or was "not about making us look bad or feel bad."

Demonstrations of the hidden curriculum by attendings is not always so overt. In a subtle but meaningful example, an attending wordlessly and without hesitation bent to pick up a small piece of garbage from the hallway floor not once, not twice, but three times in the span of a single morning on rounds. She was doing her part to make her surroundings just a little bit better and showing that anyone, regardless of rank and title, can do this, too.

Another common element of the hidden curriculum is the tendency to overuse medical investigation, including diagnostic tests. For example, local culture may sway learners to order daily blood tests for all their patients, and when asked for rationale, responses may include "it's just what we've always done" or "I thought the attending expected them." To combat these types of trends, a number of professional initiatives have been established in recent years that call for an end to wasteful spending, which amounts to an estimated $210 billion a year.[6]

Our attendings tended to view overuse of testing through the lens of how it and subsequent (potentially unnecessary) treatments would affect the patient. As we observed rounds with our attendings, we saw them modeling an attitude of "less is more," prioritizing the patient's comfort and safety over extra testing that was unnecessary or marginally useful. Indeed, superfluous tests can lead to a domino effect of untoward consequences such as higher costs, pain and discomfort, and worry from patients and family members. "Any labs?" one attending asked an intern. "We stopped the labs," was the response. "Oh, good," the attending commented, "only do things that will bring value." Another attending addressed his team: "To what end are we going to put this [patient] through that? We could increase his delirium, and I'm not certain we could find any cancer. I'm not in favor of putting him through this procedure."

Modeling Coping Skills

As teachers and physicians working in the frenetic hospital environment, our attendings must cope with frequent periods of stress and frustration, yet as role models it behooves them to maintain a calm and cool exterior. Their learners notice this. One learner recalled a time when his attending was unsatisfied with the update provided by a team member, which led to a very late night in the hospital. "He was concerned," the learner said, "but I have never seen him get angry. Never at all."

Two learners were discussing an attending. "I did not get the sense that he lost his temper by accident," said the first. "I think he used it as a tool to indicate that what was happening was not okay." The second learner replied, "Yeah, I've seen that, like when he says some particular thing has made him 'cranky.' He uses 'cranky' to add emphasis, right? But I haven't seen him . . . raise his voice."

One attending metered their frustration when a social worker who had been talking with a patient questioned the medical decisions. "I was in the team room later when I called [the social worker]," the attending told us, "I was very much aware that the team was listening. I was clearly upset, but I wasn't unprofessional. I was kind of proud of myself."

Our 18 attendings are upfront with their learners about some tough truths. They never stop reminding their teams, for example, that uncertainty is an integral part of the practice of medicine. The results of the physical examination are often ambiguous, as are the results of tests and consults with experts. Not only do experienced physicians sometimes disagree about a given diagnosis or treatment plan, but any one of the physicians may also have a different view of the matter on any given day. Imaging and other tests can deliver ambivalent results, accompanied by incomplete or inaccurate computer interpretations. Our attendings saw value in reviewing the studies directly with team members, both to confirm results and also to teach (see Figure 8.1).

As role models, how do the 18 attendings cope with the uncertainty factor? One of them described a patient who had both a bleeding tumor deposit in the head from metastatic cancer and a recent large pulmonary embolism, a blood clot in the lungs that would typically be treated with blood thinners. If the patient was given a blood thinning medication, there was a chance he could have a catastrophic hemorrhage in the brain. There was no clear "right" pathway, and each treatment strategy was fraught with risk. We asked the attending how she helped her team cope with such a situation. "You talk about the risks and benefits on both sides of the equation," she said, "and try to then be as transparent about the decision-making process as you can. We put our heads together to come up with the best plan for the patient while recognizing that this is the risk we're about to take." By bringing the learners into the discussion and sharing her own thought process, the attending models the collegial behavior that is most effective in resolving complex clinical problems and that shows that, sometimes, there is no right answer but rather, a best answer.

We frequently heard the 18 attendings acknowledging the uncertainties of medical practice. "It's a little bit of a mystery," said one. Another admitted, "Sometimes you go down a road that leads you nowhere." A current learner told us how his attending personalizes that unpredictability. "You know the typical stories they tell: nobody was able to figure it out, but then I came in and figured

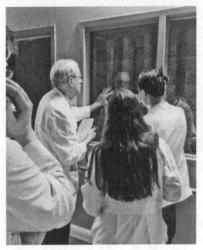 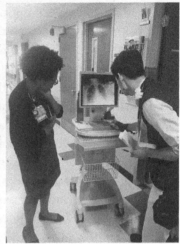

Figure 8.1 Attending and team reviewing primary studies (electrocardiogram, chest radiograph) during rounds.

it out and everything was good. Well, the stories my attending tells are mostly about the cases where he got the thing wrong. He wants to share his mistakes with you so you can learn from them." The attending was also modeling an attitude: mistakes are part and parcel of a profession that must navigate ambivalence; they are to be lamented, but there is no shame in sharing them for the growth of individuals and the good of the profession.

Where there is ambivalence, there is risk; where there is risk, there can be dire consequences. That's when attending physicians face some of their toughest role model challenges: when a patient they and their team have been caring for has an untoward outcome. They have to model the appropriate behavior not just with their teams but with the patient and the patient's family as well.

Bad outcomes can take a heavy emotional toll on individual learners and on the whole team. "I can get very emotionally invested in my patients and their families," a current learner told us, "and I know I'm going to have patients who are going to succumb to their disease. My attending really models how to deal with that, so I can in the future maybe avoid physician burnout or fatigue or lack of empathy."

We observed another attending setting an example for his team on how to cope with the recent death of one of their patients.

Attending: When we have a bad outcome, we tend to go over and over it. I spend a lot of porch time thinking about it. We should reflect on what happened but not lose our confidence. The day after he died, I sat in my truck and did a personal pep talk. You have to come in and take care of the next patient and do the best you can.

Medical student: Do you ever go to a patient's funeral?

Attending: Yes, but not for me. I go if I think it will help the family or they ask me to go. You know, if it feels like your soul has been ripped out after a bad outcome, then you've done something right. You've made that connection with the patient. My job is to build communication between all of us so we feel vested in each other and our patients.

The Joys of Medicine

A simple but immensely important method of role modeling comes down to demeanor. Portraying the joy of the profession—through humor, smiles, and a vested interest in other people (see Figure 8.2)—can inspire a team to do their best for patients and for themselves. For one attending, the most important example she sets is the evident pleasure she takes in caring for patients. "I'm a big believer in role modeling. There is a lot of joy-sucking that can happen in a hospital where people just get really entrenched on their gerbil wheels churning out patients," she said. "I think you should just stop and smell the roses, and I try to make sure we pay attention to that." A former learner summarized their reflections on a different attending.

He likes being a doctor, and you can see it when he practices. He's happy doing what he is doing. It inspires us that, yes, we will be happy just by trying to help other people by being a doctor.

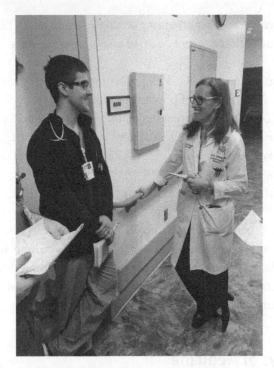

Figure 8.2 Attending outwardly demonstrating the joy of teaching with her learner.

Our attendings described the love of what they do, and perhaps none more elegantly than in this response to our question of what advice she would give to future attending physicians:

And, hopefully, to continue to model the love of patients and the love of medicine, because it's very easy to get burned out and get frustrated and to transmit that energy to your patients and to your learners . . . and to kind of have the humility of knowing what a privilege it is to do this job and, hopefully, using that as your kind of buoy. You know, recognizing that every job has its pluses and minuses, and medicine is no different but, still, whatever it is, finding whatever that joy is and what made you go into the field in the first place. And using that, especially when you are in front of your learners, I think, maybe, that might be what the biggest piece is, because they are recognizing your unconscious communication and transmitting that to their patients. I want to just make sure they are still respecting our patients, respecting each other, and above all . . . holding this job as a privilege and not just a job.

In the next chapter, we explore the role that mentors and sponsors play in the development of outstanding teaching attending physicians. We review methods that attendings may use to give and receive mentorship in order to enhance both their own teaching abilities and those of others, such as direct observation of teaching as it happens (the way we observed the 18), leadership development programs, mentoring committees, and support networks that help to publicize important achievements.

Main Points

1. Attendings hold themselves and their team members to high standards.
2. Role modeling is an important part of the teaching process and includes demonstrating how to be a diligent lifelong learner, maintaining professionalism in the face of adversity, and acknowledging the emotional toll that caring for patients can have on oneself.
3. Expressions of joy are common among the attendings, and these serve as sources of inspiration for their learners.

Further Reading

Branch WT, Jr., Kern D, Haidet P, et al. Teaching the human dimensions of care in clinical settings. JAMA 2001;286:1067–74.

    In this article, the authors describe a climate of learning that may be lacking in the teaching of humanism. They identify several strategies to overcome barriers to teaching humanism that include taking advantage of seminal events, such as demonstrating how to deliver bad news; role modeling by acting; commenting on and explaining what you have done; and using active learning skills by involving learners in tasks that require them to use humanistic skills. However, the authors point out that in order to implement these strategies, institutions must first establish a climate of humanism.

Yoon JD, Ham SA, Reddy ST, Curlin FA. Role models' influence on specialty choice for residency training: A national longitudinal study. J Grad Med Educ 2018;10:149–54.

In this five-year, longitudinal study of students from 24 US medical schools, the authors examined factors influencing medical students' choices of specialty training type. They found that interaction with a role model who displays exceptional conduct had a significant impact on the choice of specialty the student would later pursue. Medical students who had such interactions before or during medical school had higher odds of entering the same residency type as that of the role model. This prediction held true for those choosing generalist roles (i.e., primary care, pediatrics, and internal medicine), surgical roles, and radiology, ophthalmology, anesthesiology, and dermatology (ROAD) specialties. These findings indicate that institutions that train the next generation of physicians should embrace intentional use of role models to help develop students' professional identities.

Wright S, Wong A, Newill C. The impact of role models on medical students. J Gen Intern Med 1997;12:53–6.

This cross-sectional survey study examined a single cohort of medical students to examine the relationship between having a role model during medical school and the students' choices of specialty training. The authors further estimated the strength of that relationship, finding that it varied by specialty. The odds of choosing a specialty when the student had spent enough time with a given role model was 3.6 times higher for surgery, 4.6 times higher for internal medicine, 5.1 times higher for family medicine, and 12.8 times higher for pediatrics. This study identified the most important factors students consider when choosing a role model, including personality, clinical skills and competence, and teaching ability. The authors found role model research achievements and rank (academic position) were least important to students. The authors conclude that role model exposure strongly influences medical students' choices of specialty training. Identifying important factors that influence medical students' choice of role model should provide them with additional tools to select that role model.

Saint S, Fowler KE, Krein SL, et al. An academic hospitalist model to improve healthcare worker communication and learner education: Results from a quasi-experimental study at a Veterans Affairs medical center. J Hosp Med 2013;8:702–10.

In this multimodal systems redesign of one of four medical teams in a Midwestern Veterans Affairs medical center, the authors tested various approaches to improving healthcare worker communication and learner education. The authors found that the intervention team's attendings received higher teaching scores and that third-year medical students scored significantly higher on their end-of-rotation shelf exam, indicating that a focus on improving communication and enhancing learner education is possible without increasing patient length of stay or readmission rates.

9
Mentors and Sponsors

*A mentor is someone who allows you to see the hope inside
yourself.*

—Oprah Winfrey

Never have leadership, mentorship, and sponsorship been more important in healthcare. Previous chapters have alluded to the immense challenges the field faces, not the least of which are large, complex, intricate, and highly specialized healthcare teams that must work together cohesively toward the common goal of outstanding patient care. The marked rates of burnout—encompassed by depersonalization, emotional exhaustion, and decreased motivation—have contributed to lower rates of patient safety and satisfaction, and higher healthcare costs. All this in a moment in history with heightened focus on safety, quality, and the patient experience.

Why are leaders so important? Leadership has been described as "the most influential factor in shaping organizational culture."[1] Indeed, numerous articles and books have described a consistent association between effective leadership and important outcomes in the realms of safety, satisfaction, and resilience.[2-6] On the other hand, poor leadership has been noted as a potential contributor to failures of patient safety systems and higher rates of healthcare employee burnout.[7,8]

Many distinct, and sometimes overlapping, types of leadership have been described in different industries, and each is replete with its own strengths, drawbacks, and unique traits. For instance,

Teaching Inpatient Medicine. Second Edition. Nathan Houchens, Molly Harrod, and Sanjay Saint,
Oxford University Press. © Nathan Houchens, Molly Harrod, and Sanjay Saint 2023.
DOI: 10.1093/oso/9780197639023.003.0009

relational leadership (when leaders form meaningful bonds) tends to be associated with higher rates of nurse job satisfaction, lower rates of patient death, and higher rates of patient satisfaction.[9] Conversely, autocratic leadership that focuses on power differentials and hierarchy tends to stymie the culture of safety through worry, blame, and retribution for bringing important patient safety issues to the forefront or identifying issues in quality of care.[10]

Many individuals can easily and quickly recall the best leaders with whom they have worked. It's likely that they can just as rapidly identify the less-than-ideal leaders, too. Typically, effective leaders portray emotional intelligence, often described through important traits like self-awareness, self-management, social awareness, and relationship management. When leaders (even those without the formal "leader" designation) harness emotional intelligence and relationally connect with those in their group, it leads to positive outcomes.[11] However, when leaders contribute or drive negative emotions, it can lead to toxicity and poor performance.[11]

Leadership is intimately intertwined with mentorship and sponsorship.[12] From its origins in Homer's *The Odyssey*, in which Mentor serves as a guide and source of support for Telemachus,[13] mentorship has long been recognized as a key to physicians' personal and professional development. Likewise, sponsorship—active support by someone appropriately placed in the organization who has significant influence on decision-making processes or structures, and who is advocating for, protecting, and fighting for the career advancement of an individual[14]—is gaining recognition as an equally important part of growth, particularly for women and underrepresented minorities in medicine. They all complement and augment each other.

Leadership is a social activity, and thus, relationships among individuals within the group are a key variable in determining how leadership is viewed and received. While the historical concept of a leader tended to emphasize the individual person, the focus more recently has shifted to distribution or sharing of leadership across roles and responsibilities within an organization. This collective leadership style, in which many are considered leaders and the group members empower each other, has been found to be a better predictor of team performance and effectiveness when compared with more traditional vertical approaches.[15,16]

In the previous chapter, we discussed the ways in which exemplary teaching attending physicians foster a positive hidden curriculum by inspiring their learners to be their best selves. Now we turn our attention to the myriad ways in which attendings more explicitly provide and receive leadership, mentorship, and sponsorship. We describe findings from our study about mentorship and sponsorship among women and underrepresented minorities, transition to general mentorship techniques and strategies, and conclude with practical examples of mentoring and leadership curricula and programs from our own institution. We hope that these pages allow mentors in medicine to, in the words of *New York Times* best-selling author Suze Orman, "help people become more of who they already are."[17]

Mentorship and Networks of Support

Roughly equal numbers of men and women matriculate into medical schools each year, yet nearly three-quarters of senior leadership roles in healthcare organizations are filled by men.[18] This makes for a very high likelihood of cross-gender mentorships. In these situations, three practices[18] can be broadly applied to encourage the best outcome.

1. *Avoid gender scripts.* These antiquated social heuristics promote an outdated view of women as having less authority than men. They rely on archetypal roles (e.g., protector/protected) that reinforce the stereotype that women need to be "rescued." Instead, mentors can focus on identifying any latent gender-based biases (and combat them accordingly) and encouraging self-efficacy and agency as a mentee develops.
2. *Promote reciprocal learning.* Rather than relying on the staid mentor-to-mentee transfer of knowledge, mentors can focus on ways that learning can flow in both directions. For instance,

mentors can encourage female mentees to hone their own leadership style and collaboratively develop and optimize that style. Mentors may ask questions of their mentees in order to recognize and appreciate their competency and learn from their knowledge, experiences, and points of view.

3. *Be the change you want to see.* In many institutions, women may have less social capital compared to men as a result of gender biases. Thus, male mentors may spend their own capital wisely to promote gender equity. From hiring, salary, and benefits policies, to nominating women for talks, awards, and leadership positions, the male mentor often has many ways to support female mentees.[18]

During our interviews with exemplary attending physicians who self-identify as women, our research team noted the ways they described their role models and mentors and the important ways in which their careers were shaped by these key individuals. Sometimes these role models were males in authority positions—perhaps team members helping to care for patients. One of the 18 attendings told us a story about when she was a resident that highlighted the power of having her male attending physician support her in front of their patient.

When I was a resident, I had a situation where I was the resident in charge and my attending—a white male—came in and then the patient said . . . "I don't want to have a female." It wasn't for . . . reasons that would be socially acceptable. . . . And it wasn't anything we did. It wasn't that we didn't provide good care. "I just want to talk to you. You look like *you* [the male attending] should be the one who is in charge." And my attending just was like, "Excuse me? This is my team. This is the doctor in charge," and pointed to me. It was like, "She is competent. . . . She is amazing, you need to talk to her." And that feeling. . . . How empowered I felt from that was just amazing! So I try to do the same thing.

Other times, the outstanding teaching attendings would serve as role models themselves by adopting the motto made famous by the Los

Angeles Police Department in 1963: "To Protect and to Serve."[19] In essence, this is to say that female attendings, while serving patients, felt the need to protect their learners using their leadership roles. This protection often was necessary because someone was being inappropriate: harassment, discrimination, microaggressions, and other forms of biased behavior. One attending told us,

> I had very frank discussions about harassment with some now former learners while they were in our training program. You know, our institution has been great about establishing sort of a pathway that people can follow, and so it's more just sort of the encouragement and the courage to report things that they were experiencing, or they saw on behalf of colleagues. So, yeah, I think I have gotten a reputation maybe as a momma bear for some people. That's the situation people come to talk to me about in terms of how to handle [it].

The female teaching attendings we observed and interviewed took their role as mentor very seriously, particularly for other female learners. During our interview with one of the 18 attendings, we heard about the inherent connectedness felt by teams that are made up of women.

> I mean, it's great to be a role model for other women who are going through [it]. You know, I love having all-women teams. I really do. . . . There's something special about that. Like, we really bond in a way, and I think work together so well—just . . . the solidarity, I guess. It's hard to explain, but I think the role model part is nice.

Support, mentorship, and sponsorship does not just occur in the midst of inpatient clinical care rounds and in the hospital. Dedicated networks of individuals, linked through the mutual goal of supporting and promoting each other's successes and works, were sometimes mentioned in our interviews. One attending we visited shared with us the current state at her institution. She shared a story in which two physicians at her hospital received the same award at the same ceremony. One of the recipients (who happened to be a man) publicized the award, notice was sent around, and there was a lot of recognition. Yet none of the same acknowledgment and public recognition were given for the other recipient (who happened to be a woman) until someone in the hospital spoke up. Thereafter, others commented, "Oh sorry, we didn't know you were awarded also."

This attending told us that there is an entire support network of women and junior faculty who have been forged to promote each other's successes. The group, composed of female physicians and "one shy man," was established since "some people are good at self-promotion, and some are not." The attending mentioned to us that she is part of this network and that they purposefully lift each other up by sharing accomplishments and distributing and publicizing their papers and awards.

Doctors as Mentors

The similarities between the roles of doctor and mentor are marked, including an imbalance of power (for doctors, a differential of power between themselves and their patients; for mentors, between themselves and their mentees), experience, and knowledge.[20] In both positions, the doctor must keep the patient's or mentee's interests in mind. Without a deliberate approach to mentoring and a clear focus on the needs of the mentee, it is quite easy for "mentorship malpractice" to occur.[21]

Many may believe that effective mentoring can only occur with a large investment of time and energy. However, even very busy doctors can provide invaluable mentoring, even if time or location are limiting factors. Mentors may consider using alternative (i.e., virtual) methods to communicate when it is not feasible to meet in person. Any time spent with a mentee can be of benefit.

Similarly, when many people envision mentoring, they focus only on the traditional dyad (one-on-one) form, which does often involve a tremendous commitment of time and resources. Yet this is only one form of mentoring. Other mentoring roles may work better in a given situation if mentors do not have the time for the traditional role. A mentor's position may allow them to work as a coach (help with a specific issue), sponsor (help raise visibility of a mentee), or connector (help pair mentees together with other individuals or groups).[12]

Regardless of the role a mentor takes on, maintaining a steady and objective view of the mentee will help the relationship succeed. *Mindfulness* is a technique that can aid the mentor in remaining objective and being aware of the mentee's point of view. In all mentorship interactions, it is necessary for the mentor to remain nonjudgmental and supportive of the mentee while distancing themselves from their emotions.[22] Mindfulness can similarly assist the mentor in remembering that being a physician is hard work and involves overcoming many obstacles. Mentors are most helpful when keeping these ideas at the forefront of their minds.

Applying mindfulness in the context of mentorship can have other profound and positive impacts on the mentoring relationship in any form. As one of us wrote before, mentors who regularly practice mindfulness can "become selfless, compassionate, and authentic," leading to a more trusting mentor–mentee relationship that can allow the mentee to attempt higher-risk, higher-reward projects.[22] Mindfulness in mentoring can be undertaken with just five simple steps,[22] herein written with you, the mentor, in mind:

1. *Start with yourself.* An understanding of why you want to mentor will provide a solid basis from which to begin. Asking yourself if you are providing what your mentee needs, if you are growing from the relationship, and if you can accept both success and failure in your mentees will ensure that your approach originates from a true motivation.

2. *Put yourself in their shoes.* After many years of mentoring, one can forget the absolute requirement to be compassionate and empathic in the mentoring relationship. A kind approach coupled with constructive and actionable advice will foster a nurturing, rather than punitive, environment. As in many aspects of life, the golden rule of treating a mentee how the mentor would want to be treated is the best approach.

3. *Practice slowing down.* Mindfulness is about being present, and mindful mentors know that the busy lives they and their mentees lead can easily make them rush through tasks and interactions. Staying present during mentor–mentee encounters allows the mentor to be less judgmental and more curious, which may enhance emotional intelligence and lead to identification and resolution of hard-to-discuss, but critical, issues.

4. *Be grateful.* Recognize that mentoring is a gift in that, as a mentor, you are helping shape the next generation of physicians. Being aware of and expressing gratitude has multiple benefits: it is positively associated with happiness, it engenders in the mentee a sense of being valued (which often leads to harder and more effective work and more receptivity to criticism), and it is infectious (spreading gratitude from you, the mentee, and beyond).

5. *Embrace selflessness.* The ultimate goal for the mentor is to help their mentee become the best version of themself. This means guiding (not commanding), making suggestions (not leading), and helping revise work (not rejecting it). When the mentee succeeds, the mentor deflects praise to them. When there are problems, the mentor accepts them as their own difficulties. These approaches encapsulate selflessness in mentoring.[22]

Mentorship Roles and Archetypes

The traditional longitudinal mentor–mentee one-on-one dyad is just one of several important types of mentoring that can help mentees succeed. Indeed, with a lack of sufficient numbers of mentors, having alternative paths to share and gain knowledge is critical to the future of mentoring. While we have thus far focused primarily on the traditional mentor, it is worth noting that there are four archetypes of mentorship: (1) the traditional mentor, (2) the coach, (3) the sponsor, and (4) the connector.[12]

Coaches focus on a particular problem a mentee may have or help the mentee develop a specific skillset, so these relationships tend to be more ephemeral. An interesting advantage of the coaching approach is that it can be done in group settings, such that helping address specific problems or gain specific skills can be done in a more efficient manner.

Sponsors, as defined previously, tend to focus on more strategic goals of mentoring, either in a specific dyad or in the larger context of a mentoring program. They help make mentees more visible by recommending them to give a high-profile talk, publicizing their achievements, and suggesting they serve on panels or as a study section reviewer. Sponsors are unique because they are often invisible to the mentee, working behind the scenes to grow the field and develop talent.

The last archetype is the *connector*, a person who has an extensive network and substantial social and political capital built up from a long, successful career of their own. Since connectors focus on the entire field, their motivation is rooted in a legacy. As current and future mentors, it is crucial to understand what role a mentee expects of you or needs you to perform.[12]

Mentoring Millennials

Today, most students entering medical schools and residency training are part of the "Millennial" generation: those individuals born between 1980 and 2000.[23] Unlike perhaps any previous intergenerational shift, Millennials have had a distinct influence in medicine. This generation values rapid information and groupthink due to enhanced social networking and a technologically connected global culture.[23] The hierarchical structure of medicine embraced by past generations is of lesser concern to many Millennials and can lead to conflict between more senior faculty and Millennial learners and mentees. Given these (at times) conflicting values and the hierarchical nature of historical teacher–learner education, learning and the mentoring relationship may be affected.

Rather than dwell on the conflicts this may cause, it is worthwhile to recognize the myths about the Millennial generation that should be clarified or dispelled so that the most inclusive and effective teaching and mentoring environment can be established. Other generations may have misconceptions that Millennials are impatient, entitled, lazy, or needy. These negative perceptions boil down to a difference in generational values and methods of work. Millennial individuals frequently value efficiency and engagement through quickly accessible data and collaboration. They are more often motivated by purpose, meaning in their work, and skill, instead of the traditional advancement metrics or accomplishments by "time-in-rank."[23,24] Millennials have also grown up during a time of greater social consciousness and typically value diversity and autonomy rather than uniformity. To best mentor individuals belonging to this group, it is important to embrace innovation, purpose, autonomy, diversity, and social networking and avoid inertia, busywork, isolation, and strict hierarchy.[23]

Intergenerational differences should be acknowledged and addressed to achieve a productive learning and mentoring relationship. Members of all generations contribute to the immense value of a diverse team. And while the methods may change between generations, all physicians seek professional advancement, collaboration, and purpose.

Direct Observations and Feedback

In their 2008 review of the literature on good clinical teachers in medicine, Sutkin and colleagues noted that "two-thirds of characteristics of outstanding clinical teachers are 'noncognitive,'" and that "perhaps what makes a clinical educator truly great depends ... more on inherent, relationship-based, noncognitive attributes."[25] Put another way, just as cultivating connections with patients is important for high-quality patient care, forming bonds with learners is important for high-quality teaching. It is not just about *what* the teacher knows, but *how* the teacher asks questions, communicates their thoughts, and facilitates discussion.

Nowhere did we find bonds formed with learners and enviable communication styles more than with our 18 exemplary attendings. By reviewing interviews and field notes from our own observations of them, we culled quotes, techniques, and strategies to those core behaviors that, when used with teams, contribute to optimal learning environments. Indeed, these core behaviors form the foundation of this book.

In an effort to further spread the word about all the evidence-based effective behaviors and techniques the 18 brought each day to inpatient rounds, our institution established the *DOCTOR program*, which stands for Direct Observations of Clinical Teaching On Rounds. This program is one form of the coaching archetype described previously and is geared toward clinician educators (e.g., teaching attendings both junior and senior, fellows, and chief medical residents). The program involves in-person observations of teaching techniques in authentic clinical environments. The observer, a clinician familiar with the foundational research on the 18 outstanding teaching attendings and effective teaching in general, accompanies a clinical team on rounds; focuses on discrete, tangible, observable behaviors from the clinician educator; and records their findings on an observation checklist (see Figure 9.1). The checklist includes behaviors that exhibit interactional skills with team members, such as regular use of first names and demonstrating interest in learners as people; teaching skills, shown by probing learner understanding and facilitating teaching points; skills with patients, such as building rapport and demonstrating respect through social interaction; and effective education and planning, such as use of reflective listening and avoiding medical jargon. After rounds, there is a session of one-on-one dedicated feedback between the observer and clinician educator on the teaching approach, including what about the clinician educator's approach was effective and strategies to improve it. The goal is for this program to be a form of the aforementioned *reciprocal learning*, a two-way street. That is, the observer and clinician educator switch roles so they can observe each other

DOCTOR PROGRAM OBSERVATION FORM

Clinician-Educator _____ Observer _____ Date _____ Total Time _____

INTERACTIONS WITH TEAM	Frequency CIRCLE ONE: 1=Never, 3= 50% of the time, 5=All of the time	EXAMPLES, NOTES (SPECIFIC examples of actions, behaviors, phrases, and nonverbals)
Uses learners' first names regularly	1 2 3 4 5 N/A	
Demonstrates interest in learners as people (e.g. career goals, hobbies, activities on days off)	1 2 3 4 5 N/A	
Shows vulnerability by admitting own mistakes and uncertainty	1 2 3 4 5 N/A	
Seeks input from other healthcare professionals and models inter-professional communication (e.g. with bedside nurse or pharmacist/pharmacy student)	1 2 3 4 5 N/A	
Avoids interrupting learners	1 2 3 4 5 N/A	
Shows respect for learners' time (e.g. flexibility with rounds, allowing senior resident to choose rounding order, split rounds, see patients alone if needed)	Yes No N/A	

TEACHING	Frequency CIRCLE ONE: 1=Never, 3= 50% of the time, 5=All of the time	EXAMPLES, NOTES (SPECIFIC examples of actions, behaviors, phrases, and nonverbals)
Invites learners to provide opinions, ideas, and suggestions	1 2 3 4 5 N/A	
Asks questions to probe learner understanding (e.g. think aloud, give rationale for decisions)	1 2 3 4 5 N/A	
Facilitates at least one teaching point per patient	1 2 3 4 5 N/A	
Recommends or provides at least one learning resource based on current patients (e.g. article, guideline, handout, visual aid)	Yes No N/A	
Tailors questions to learners' educational levels, knowledge, experience, and career goals	1 2 3 4 5 N/A	
Summarizes key points of the discussion on rounds, when relevant.	1 2 3 4 5 N/A	

Figure 9.1 Direct Observations of Clinical Teaching On Rounds (DOCTOR) Program Observation Checklist.

PATIENT - RAPPORT AND RESPECT	Frequency CIRCLE ONE: 1=Never, 3= 50% of the time; 5=All of the time	EXAMPLES, NOTES (SPECIFIC examples of actions, behaviors, phrases, and nonverbals)
Greets patient in respectful way (e.g. knocks/inquires, greets warmly by name, handshake)	1 2 3 4 5 N/A	
Makes introductions and describes roles	1 2 3 4 5 N/A	
Uses effective nonverbal communication (e.g. sits or kneels at patient's eye level, maintains eye contact)	1 2 3 4 5 N/A	
Builds rapport (e.g. by making a social comment, engaging in humanistic/non-medical conversation)	1 2 3 4 5 N/A	
Shows respect during examination (e.g. asks permission to perform physical exam; protects patient's modesty and attends to comfort; assists patient in changing positions; closes door or curtain)	1 2 3 4 5 N/A	

PATIENT – EDUCATION AND PLANNING	Frequency CIRCLE ONE: 1=Never, 3= 50% of the time; 5=All of the time	EXAMPLES, NOTES (SPECIFIC examples of actions, behaviors, phrases, and nonverbals)
Uses reflective listening skills to demonstrate understanding (e.g. acknowledgement responses)	1 2 3 4 5 N/A	
Summarizes key points using an effective method of communication for the patient (e.g. visual aids, analogies)	1 2 3 4 5 N/A	
Avoids medical jargon or explains words' meanings	1 2 3 4 5 N/A	
Ensures patient/family understanding (e.g. teach-back, ask what questions/concerns can be addressed)	1 2 3 4 5 N/A	

Figure 9.1 Continued

and provide feedback, perhaps learn new strategies, and expand their clinical teaching skills.

The DOCTOR program has been instrumental in bidirectional mentorship at our institution. To date, according to our internal data, nearly 90% of all participants indicated that they would make at least one change to their rounding or teaching style as a result of the program. One participant commented, "By watching others, it brings about self-reflection as to one's own style and techniques. Made me more self-aware of some of my weaknesses."

Leadership Development for All Healthcare Employees

Given the importance of leadership to organizations like hospitals and healthcare systems and leadership development as an avenue with which to build these skills, our institution founded the Fueling Leadership in Yourself or *FLY program*.[26] FLY was established on the concept that all levels of healthcare workers, including those providing direct care to patients, may benefit from leadership development. Our goal was to invigorate teamwork, or rather a culture of collaboration, within our service and ultimately elevate autonomy in everyone's daily work.

We intentionally invited a diverse group of healthcare employees from different departments, including teaching attending physicians, to build peer networks together while also learning about and practicing collective leadership skills. This group was comprised of individuals from various roles on the healthcare team. As a part of the program, we provided exposure to key mentors within the facility (chief of medicine, health behavior coordinator, industrial engineer within the systems redesign program, inpatient care physician), individuals identified as leaders who have specific enthusiasm and expertise in a variety of leadership domains.

Content areas were chosen carefully to be universally applicable to everyone, regardless of the individual's specific role on the team or within the department or system (e.g., the art and science of leadership, mindfulness techniques to empower the self and others in the workplace, quality improvement strategies to improve daily work, and effective communication principles in healthcare environments). The program used a variety of learning styles with hierarchy-flattening, interactive exercises so that all participants felt included with their preferred learning styles. We elected to keep the series of four one-hour sessions short and limited so that the program could be expanded to other services if desired.

The individuals who have participated in the FLY series thus far have comprised six unique role types and hailed from eight distinct services, sections, or work units in the hospital. Very few participants had a specific or formal leadership role. Self-reported outcomes indicated that participants significantly increased their knowledge of leadership techniques, were highly satisfied with and would recommend the series, and found leadership principles applicable to their daily work. Some representative quotes from participants included the following:

- "I enjoyed the sessions; they were all different. I also found the references to books helpful for resources."
- "The interactive exercises were the best, the way we utilized/experienced what we were discussing."
- "Highlights: group activities, interaction, meeting the leaders in the institution, enjoyed lunches."

Structured Mentorship Through Committees

One key to success in career advancement and personal and professional satisfaction is individualized mentorship. This is most commonly found—and indeed expected—for physicians on the research track (also called *instructional* or *tenure track* at some institutions) who are often working on grant applications and projects. Yet the principles and benefits of this structure of mentorship are broadly applicable to any type of physician, including those on the clinical track—those physicians who primarily engage in direct patient care and teaching. Importantly, for many who choose to leave the field of medicine, lack of mentorship is seen as an important contributor to dissatisfaction.

Our institution has shown its commitment to mentorship for all clinical track faculty by establishing the Clinician Mentoring Program. For any junior faculty member, a mentoring committee is established. These committees are comprised of between three and six committee members and one committee chair, chosen by the mentee and trusted advisors. The committee chair is often a section or division chief. Other mentors who serve on the committee—such as leaders in the system, research, quality improvement, education, policy, or any domain in which the mentee is interested—are also invaluable members.

For mentees in the Clinician Mentoring Program, mentoring committee meetings occur once or twice per year, for one hour at a time, held in person or virtually. There is a lot of preparation to ensure that these meetings are useful. A project manager arranges, coordinates, and assists with all meeting materials, including distributing an updated copy of the mentee's curriculum vitae (CV) to all members of the committee for review before the meeting. The mentee is expected to be familiar with key resources, such as general guidance for effective menteeship[27] and clinical track promotional information and criteria for the academic institution. During meetings, the mentee and committee chair guide a conversation that spans the mentee's short-, mid-, and long-term goals; an assessment of personal and professional satisfaction with the mentee's current role; updates in the key areas in which the mentee is spending time; and feedback on how the committee can most effectively mentor and sponsor the mentee.

At the conclusion of each mentoring committee meeting, we collect feedback using a standardized Mentoring Meeting Assessment Tool (see Figure 9.2). This Likert scale–based survey of all participants, including mentee, chair, and mentoring committee members, elicits information on logistics of the meeting (e.g., started on time, CV was distributed beforehand, it was a good use of time), perceptions of how feedback was received, clarity of next steps, assessment of progress since the last meeting, and impacts of the mentoring program on satisfaction and burnout.

Mentoring Meeting Assessment Tool (MMAT)

1. Please enter your name _____

2. Please enter your role (select only one option)
   - ☐ Mentee
   - ☐ Mentoring committee chair
   - ☐ Mentoring committee member

3. Please enter the mentee's name (MENTORS ONLY) _____

4. Please enter the date of the meeting (MENTEES ONLY)_____

5. Mentee's CV was sent to all mentors before the meeting (MENTORS ONLY)
   - ☐ Yes
   - ☐ No

6. The meeting began on time
   - ☐ Yes
   - ☐ No

7. Sufficient time was allotted for the meeting
   - ☐ Strongly agree
   - ☐ Agree
   - ☐ Neither agree nor disagree
   - ☐ Disagree
   - ☐ Strongly disagree

8. Overall, the meeting was an effective use of my time
   - ☐ Strongly agree
   - ☐ Agree
   - ☐ Neither agree nor disagree
   - ☐ Disagree
   - ☐ Strongly disagree

9. I discussed _____ action items I wanted to during the meeting (MENTEE ONLY)
   - ☐ All
   - ☐ Most
   - ☐ Some
   - ☐ Few
   - ☐ No

10. I felt comfortable raising issues with mentors (MENTEE ONLY)
    - ☐ Strongly agree
    - ☐ Agree
    - ☐ Neither agree nor disagree
    - ☐ Disagree
    - ☐ Strongly disagree

11. Feedback given by mentors was specific, actionable, and focused on how to improve (MENTEE ONLY)
    - ☐ Strongly agree
    - ☐ Agree
    - ☐ Neither agree nor disagree
    - ☐ Disagree
    - ☐ Strongly disagree

Figure 9.2 Mentoring Meeting Assessment Tool.

12. Feedback given by mentors was received in a positive manner by mentee (MENTORS ONLY)
- ☐ Strongly agree
- ☐ Agree
- ☐ Neither agree nor disagree
- ☐ Disagree
- ☐ Strongly disagree

13. I trust that my mentors are committed to my professional success (MENTEE ONLY)
- ☐ Strongly agree
- ☐ Agree
- ☐ Neither agree nor disagree
- ☐ Disagree
- ☐ Strongly disagree

14. My mentors are helping me set and achieve career goals (MENTEE ONLY)
- ☐ Strongly agree
- ☐ Agree
- ☐ Neither agree nor disagree
- ☐ Disagree
- ☐ Strongly disagree

15. At the end of the meeting, next steps were clear (i.e., who is doing what by when)
- ☐ Strongly agree
- ☐ Agree
- ☐ Neither agree nor disagree
- ☐ Disagree
- ☐ Strongly disagree

16. Overall, this mentoring program has increased my level of satisfaction with my work
- ☐ Strongly agree
- ☐ Agree
- ☐ Neither agree nor disagree
- ☐ Disagree
- ☐ Strongly disagree

17. Overall, this mentoring program has reduced my level of burnout (e.g., exhaustion, depersonalization, and/or reduced achievement) from my work
- ☐ Strongly agree
- ☐ Agree
- ☐ Neither agree nor disagree
- ☐ Disagree
- ☐ Strongly disagree

Please provide additional comments:

Figure 9.2 Continued

To date, the program is comprised of 21 individual mentees for whom 42 distinct meetings have been conducted. Internal data show the program's positive impacts on both mentors and mentees. With respect to mentors, 98% of responses agreed ("agree" or "strongly agree") that committee meetings were an effective use of their time, 99% agreed that feedback provided was received by the mentee in a positive manner, 83% agreed that the mentoring program increased their work satisfaction, and 57% agreed that the program reduced their level of burnout. With respect to mentees, 98% of responses agreed that committee meetings were an effective use of their time and that they were comfortable raising issues with their mentors, 88% agreed that the mentoring program increased their work satisfaction, and 58% agreed that the program reduced their level of burnout. All mentee responses agreed that feedback provided was specific, actionable, and focused on how to improve; that they trust that mentors are committed to their professional success; and that mentors are helping them set and achieve career goals.

In the next chapter, we shift gears from how physicians serve as leaders and provide and receive guidance to the techniques they use to effectively communicate. We explore the fundamental building blocks of relationship-centered communication in healthcare and how exemplary teaching attendings use these skills to connect with patients, foster meaningful relationships, and make space for sacred moments.

Main Points

1. Leadership, mentorship, and sponsorship are unique entities but are closely intertwined. In these contexts, mentorship entails a mentor providing advice, feedback, coaching, or connection to a mentee, whereas sponsorship encompasses active support by an established sponsor who is advocating for and enhancing visibility of the individual.

2. Whether through formal, structured mentoring committees or more informal mentoring relationships, physicians frequently serve as guides for mentees to assist with professional growth. When mentors apply principles of mindfulness and recognize what the mentee hopes for or expects from the mentor, it can result in meaningful and effective interactions.

3. A variety of different formal structures within institutions may help to elevate mentorship. These could include bidirectional observation of teaching techniques with dedicated feedback, leadership development series, or physician mentoring committee programs.

Further Reading

Chopra V, Edelson DP, Saint S. Mentorship malpractice. JAMA 2016;315:1453–4.
Mentoring can be a very demanding enterprise at times. When combined with the clinical, administrative, and personal obligations physicians have, it is only natural that there will be times when mentoring does not go as well as hoped due to relatively minor lapses. When a mentor crosses a line and puts the mentee's career at risk, the authors of this paper term this "mentorship malpractice." A poor or unethical mentor can permanently damage a mentee's career. This paper details two forms of mentorship malpractice (active and passive), providing six total types that can occur in toxic mentoring relationships while also offering mentees advice on how they can be complicit (or not) in their own sabotage. The types of mentorship malpractice described are the Hijacker, Exploiter, Possessor, Bottleneck, Country Clubber, and World Traveler.

Chopra V, Vaughn V, Saint S. The Mentoring Guide: Helping Mentors and Mentees Succeed. Ann Arbor, MI: Michigan Publishing Services; 2019.
This book is a resource for mentors and mentees alike, summarizing an array of stories and data that provide concrete and practical advice on how to get the most out of each mentoring relationship. From starting as a mentee to the importance of being a good mentor, this book addresses common pitfalls and challenges and aims to help build long-term, productive, and successful mentoring relationships.

Levy BD, Katz JT, Wolf MA, Sillman JS, Handin RI, Dzau VJ. An initiative in mentoring to promote residents' and faculty members' careers. Acad Med 2004;79:845–50.

This instructive article details one approach to the problem of building a robust mentoring program within a busy, academic residency program. Since residency is such a crucial and formative point in a physician's career, it is often a time when spontaneous mentoring relationships develop. These mentoring relationships provide valuable support to residents in many of the ways that supervisors or preceptors do, with one notable difference. The most sought-after mentors are those who exist outside of the resident's performance evaluation in the residency program. Unfortunately, at many institutions, these mentoring efforts go unrewarded (in both dollars and praise). The authors formulated a mentoring program that matched residents and faculty. Findings included self-assessments of residents' mentoring needs, a list of traits of an effective mentor, and feedback from participants post-program. The feedback indicated a true need for such formalized programs, while a substantial proportion indicated that their mentors were both helpful and available. This program ensured all residents had a mentor, provided structure for mentor–mentee interactions, and increased recognition for the mentoring efforts of the faculty.

Saint S, Chopra V. Thirty Rules for Healthcare Leaders. Ann Arbor, MI: Michigan Publishing Services; 2019.

This book provides pithy pearls of wisdom specifically geared toward leaders and leaders-to-be in healthcare. Intended for all roles in healthcare—regardless of title or experience—and designed for the time-pressured individual, each rule provides practical advice that can be put to use immediately.

10

The Stories We Share

There is no greater agony than bearing an untold story inside you.

—Maya Angelou

The ways in which a physician and patient interact have meaningful effects on the relationship and on important health outcomes. The foundation of an effective relationship centers on mutual trust and respect. Building rapport in the hospital can be challenging since many physicians have not previously met the patient and family members and are often doing so during moments of duress and stress. Yet rapidly building rapport is critical to ensuring high-quality care and good patient outcomes.

Effective communication has a multitude of beneficial effects for both patients and healthcare providers. Patients enjoy improved health, such as better control of blood glucose in those with diabetes mellitus.[1,2] They more often recall medical information and understand it better. They more often have enhanced satisfaction and trust with their healthcare providers, adherence to medical treatment plans, and overall health status and quality of life.[3-7]

Physicians and other providers note improvements in diagnostic accuracy, efficiency, satisfaction, and engagement.[8-12] Unwanted outcomes, like high costs of care and malpractice claims, decrease with effective communication.[2,8,13] With the challenges of burnout and compassion fatigue on the minds of physicians and healthcare systems, it is even more important that relationship-centered communication can lead to improvements in both areas.[14] Given

Teaching Inpatient Medicine. Second Edition. Nathan Houchens, Molly Harrod, and Sanjay Saint, Oxford University Press. © Nathan Houchens, Molly Harrod, and Sanjay Saint 2023. DOI: 10.1093/oso/9780197639023.003.0010

the challenges of modern medicine described in prior chapters, never has there been a better time to invest in relationships and communication.

During a typical conversation, our attendings used dialogue—rather than monologue—to first inquire about the patient's current understanding of the condition; then share details about the illness, test results, and treatment plan in short chunks and without the use of medical terms and jargon; and finally check in with the patient to determine their updated understanding. When patients feel their physicians care, they are more likely to divulge personal information, engage in recommended testing and treatment plans, and have improved health. They may also be more inclined to share important feedback about the team.

This chapter discusses the importance of relationship-centered communication in healthcare, key elements of effective communication, empathic responses, and the sacred moments shared between patient and provider. The goal is to equip attendings—and all healthcare providers, really—with skills so that they may better elicit the untold story from their patients.

Building Blocks of Effective Communication

For several decades, much has been written about relationship-centered communication, and the various elements that make up this type of communication have been broken into discrete series of skills and behaviors. These techniques have been combined to establish models of communication which can then be used in teaching and learning in the hospital. In 1999, experts in healthcare communication gathered to formulate and crystallize important concepts in communication. The result was known as the *Kalamazoo consensus statement*,[15] a framework of critical communication skills.

Since that time, a variety of communication models have been derived, although nearly all share common features. The basic building blocks of effective communication mirror the series of events that occur during a typical encounter in the hospital. These include opening skills, interviewing and examination skills, and closing skills. Nonverbal communication and demonstrations of empathy also play important roles in building connections between people.

Opening Skills

Our attendings consistently convey value and respect through a variety of opening skills—starting with a warm and pleasant greeting. With a smile and a handshake or a wave, attendings set the tone for positive interactions. Many attendings would introduce themselves and their team members, especially if it was a larger team or the first time meeting each other.

Attendings were sure to minimize distractions during their discussions with patients. In one exchange, we witnessed an attending ask, "Is it okay if we turn down your television volume?" When the patient responded with, "You can go ahead and turn it off," the attending responded empathically with, "Actually, it can be hard to find the channel you were on, so I'll just turn it down for now."

On multiple occasions, our exemplary 18 attendings would begin the conversation with a nonmedical topic to quickly build rapport, a practice that has gained traction in the peer-reviewed literature.[16,17] Sometimes this was in response to cues in the room. For instance, "I like your hat." When looking at an empty breakfast tray, one attending exclaimed to the patient with a smile, "Well, you didn't like *any* of that!" An attentive attending noticed flowers in the room and commented, "Your wife brought more roses. They are gorgeous." This same attending with the very next patient inquired, "Is that your puppy dog?" after seeing a patient's family member with a dog's face on their T-shirt.

At times, these nonmedical comments would be focused on who the patient is as a person, what they do, and what they enjoy doing. With a pat on the hand, one attending remarked to a patient, "You're a fencer, are you? You can teach our senior resident a thing or two." In one exchange, another attending had several exploratory questions for the patient, including "Where are you from?" When the patient reported they were born in that very same town, more questions flowed: "Are you a [hospital name] baby? Where did you go to school? What kind of work do you do? How long have you not been working?" Yet another attending, again with her hand on the patient's hand: "Tell me about your family. They are in Mexico, right?"

Sometimes rapport-building is based on events in the patient's life. Our attendings would often be completely attuned to these fine details. For instance, upon entering the patient's room, the attending happily remarked "Happy belated birthday! I heard there were good muffins to celebrate the occasion."

Interviewing and Examination Skills

When interviewing a patient, our attendings remember the importance of various interview and physical examination techniques: eliciting the patient's narrative by starting with open-ended questions, encouraging further dialogue, using reflective listening, and summarizing to check for accuracy.

Our teaching attendings would avoid interrupting the patient and let them share whatever they wished. They used reflective listening to demonstrate they had heard—and really understood—the patient. In one encounter, when a family member mentioned that the patient was not receiving medication as he should have been, the attending responded, "I heard about that. This is definitely a concern of ours as well. I can appreciate why this would be frustrating. We want what's best for your father, and we appreciate you bringing this to our attention." In another encounter, when a patient was describing sudden relief from diarrhea to the point of constipation, the attending chuckled, "It's all or nothing with bowel movements, huh?" Last, as a patient was describing what helped them to avoid alcohol, the attending reflected, "It seems like your work is important to keep away from drinking."

Rapport-building and kindness allow the patient to feel comfortable disclosing personal and intimate details. Our attendings helped to elicit the patient narrative and perspective with questions like, "What makes you nervous?" In one encounter, a patient and her daughter were exchanging looks. With a laugh, the attending said "You're giving each other a look. I wonder what you're thinking?"

Understanding the patient's viewpoints on the proposed plan of care can help to determine if they will follow through with it or not. Take this empathic example: "I think your daughter just wants for you what anyone wants for themselves. And sometimes that means you may need some extra help. When people say that to you, they mean going to live someplace else. How do you feel about that?"

And finally, attendings would, at times, make the patient's perspective an explicit teaching point. One attending said to the patient: "What do you think is going on?" The patient responded, "I was worried, because my dad had those kinds of symptoms and it ended up being a stroke." The attending turned to the team and mentioned, "Team, that's the explanatory model. He thinks he may have had a stroke." She then proceeded with questions to the patient to assess thinking and orientation.

Our attendings treated all patients with dignity and respect at all times. This was never more apparent than during the physical examination. One attending asked his other team members to close the door and draw the curtain during any physical exam maneuvers. Others were more explicit about this with patients themselves. "I'll keep you modest," one attending mentioned to her patient, "but I'd like to examine your stomach if that's okay."

Closing Skills

Closing skills help to wrap up the discussion and allow an opportunity to assess for patient understanding of the plan for the day and what to expect next. A critical element in this domain is avoiding or explaining any instances of medical jargon. In many situations, teams would use words and phrases that are common among healthcare providers but unlikely to be understood by non-clinicians in the room. If that occurred, the attendings would invariably mention, "Let me tell you what we were just talking about" to explain the unfamiliar words. In another example, an attending turns to her team members who had been discussing the patient's condition in the room using medical language saying, "Why don't we translate this for these fine folks?"

Attendings would always check in with the patients after discussing the plan to address any lingering questions. "What concerns do you have? What do you still need for today? Are you warm enough? Thirsty?" Attendings would show interest in loved ones who would come to visit the patient in the hospital. "Who's coming to visit you here today?" In the next chapter, we examine *teach-back*, a technique to elucidate a patient's understanding of what has been discussed in more detail.

Attendings role-model trying to accommodate as many aspects of the patient's normal life as possible. In one example, a family member reported that the patient normally sits in his wheelchair at home. The attending responded, "He's more than welcome to do that here in the hospital as well." Attendings would return the room to the condition it was in before the team came in. They would turn the TV back on (or volume back up), put the bed's side rails back up, and put the patient's socks back on. On their way out, our attendings would often share a bit of cheerful positivity: "You're looking great!" or "we gotta stop meeting like this!"

Nonverbal Communication

How a physician communicates is often just as important as *what* is communicated. Our exemplary attendings employ different methods of nonverbal communication during their interactions. These include body postures—like kneeling, sitting, or leaning at the edge of the bed—to get at the patient's eye level. They would also use therapeutic touch liberally, including touching the shoulder during auscultation of the lungs and even encouraging the patient to hold their hand during elements of the physical exam.

Nonverbal communication also includes the physician's clothing. One attending makes it explicit in her expectations of learners to dress neatly and professionally. Many teams wear white coats when seeing patients, since the white coat is often seen as a symbol of the profession and can foster trust and confidence in patients. There is a wealth of literature describing patient preferences for different types of physician attire, and, perhaps not surprisingly, what patients prefer depends on what kind of care they are receiving, the care setting and geographic region, and factors specific to the patient, such as their age.[18,19] While one physician's choice of attire will not satisfy every single patient's preference, choosing dress that helps to foster trust and respect is a good practice.

Empathy

There is perhaps no greater way to connect with another person than through demonstrations of empathy. As mentioned in a prior chapter, literature has shown that there is a sharp decline in empathy during clinical rotations in medical school training.[20] Our 18 attendings vehemently fight back against empathy decline by role modeling outstanding empathic skills with their patients. Our attendings recognized that being in the hospital is hard, distressing, painful, and anxiety-provoking. They sought to ease suffering through their words. This could take the form of respect, such as when one attending told a family member, "It's very nice that [the patient] has such an attentive family."

Other times, attendings worked to support the individuals under their care. As a patient's wife was expressing guilt about not bringing the patient in sooner when he began to notice leg weakness and involuntary movements, the attending, with a hand on her shoulder, said, "This would have happened regardless, if you were here in the hospital or not." His wife, distraught with sadness, was further comforted by the attending who put her arm around her shoulder. After a moment of silence, the attending continued, "What would he tell us if he could hear and understand everything we're saying?" With tears in her eyes, his wife responded, "I think he'd say he's totally worn down."

Sometimes simple positivity and appreciation were all that were needed in the moment. For instance, one attending remarked to a family member, "The palliative care team is really looking forward to continue to care for him." And last, "Thanks for your patience as we work to make you feel better."

Sacred Moments

Connecting with patients helps provide physicians with purpose and meaning in their work. Likewise, connecting with physicians enhances trust and healthcare outcomes for patients. *Sacred moments*, a spiritual phenomenon well described by researchers in psychotherapy, are short events in which the patient and provider experience a sense of feeling "interconnected, transcendent, and boundless."[21] These moments are highly memorable and have been described as if time stood still.[22] There is a sense of joy, peace, and empathy that then follows. They have been described as extraordinary moments in which all distractions seem to melt away and in which the person feels blessed. These moments arise out of what some call "sudden intimacies" with strangers—those moments "when the human barrier cracks open to reveal what is most secret and inarticulate." Indeed, according to some, "this is the physician's privilege: to be lifted out of the dross of common days in order to experience such clarity of feeling."[23]

Communication that centers on relationships, that seeks to explore the lived experience of the other, that is filled with dignity, hope, and gratitude, works to create environments in which sacred moments can occur.[24]

While not specifically described as a sacred moment, our team witnessed an encounter that perhaps could be described in this way. An attending and her team entered a patient's room. The patient had been grappling with alcohol withdrawal and substance use disorder and had been in the hospital for this in the past. He was clinically improved. They made introductions.

Attending: We have a big posse today. I'd like to turn off your TV so I can hear you. . . . How are you feeling today? What concerns do you have?

Patient: Life is scary, you know. This is why I drink.

Attending: Yeah, I hear you. You took a really brave step by coming in. Our job is to get you through this life-threatening piece. I know you've been at Salvation Army before. There are a lot of kind people there. . . . Tell me this, were you regularly seeing a psychiatrist or psychologist? [They discuss prior treatments and providers].

Attending: Your insight is amazing. You've done this before. Sobriety is for those who want it. [She conducts elements of the physical examination with a hand on his shoulder] You're definitely less tremulous today. . . . This team of doctors is taking care of a lot of patients who drink or use drugs. What would be your advice about those struggling with addiction?

Patient: [After a brief pause, to learners] Please understand how hard this is for me and for those others.

Attending: [With a handshake] Good luck to you, and congratulations with your sobriety. The very best is yet to come.

The following chapter continues the themes of empathy and communication by exploring attendings' care for patients in the sacred space of their hospital room. Through words and actions, the attendings attempt to meet both the physical and emotional needs of their patient to help facilitate full healing. In this way, attendings set a standard that learners may follow throughout their careers. "He was always very gentle with patients," a former learner said of one attending, "and he took the time to explain things. And I think that really helped shape who I am, because that's something, if you don't see it, you don't necessarily know that it matters. And I got to see it."

Main Points

1. Attendings use a variety of fundamental communication skills (opening, interviewing and examination, and closing skills) to form connections. Through their words and actions, they build rapport with patients and their family members and make space for sacred moments.

2. One way to form a bond quickly is through conversing about nonmedical topics. Attendings frequently explore the lived experiences of their patients.

3. Body posture and mannerisms, therapeutic touch, and clothing are important forms of nonverbal communication that can have just as much of an impact on the patient–physician relationship as verbal communication.

Further Reading

Wolpaw DR, Shapiro D. The virtues of irrelevance. N Engl J Med 2014;370:1283–5.

In many ways, our modern societies have created strain and distrust in the patient–provider relationship. Systems have made it difficult for providers and patients to connect in a meaningful and human way by always demanding more from providers and reducing time spent with the patient. This piece from the *New England Journal of Medicine* talks about one way to reintroduce connection: irrelevance. Think of this concept as akin to small talk, which provides a means to build social interactions and can be used to learn important details about the person the provider is treating. This article identifies four main ways in which engaging in this sort of irrelevant conversation with a patient can improve relations. First, this act signals to the patient that the provider sees them as an individual whose lived experience is unique and valued. Next, it helps to connect through discovery of shared experiences that allow for connection on a more personal level (despite real or perceived differences in knowledge and power). In addition, requesting and recalling specific details about a patient demonstrates that the provider is paying attention, which many patients find comforting. Finally, it shows that the provider wants to have open communication with the patient, which can contribute to higher satisfaction.

Fitzgerald FT. Curiosity. Ann Intern Med 1999;130:70–2.

For some time, a common patient concern has been an apparent lack of compassion on the part of healthcare workers. Some physicians, particularly, have gained a reputation as cold and distant: "insensitive, mechanistic, technocratic, inhumane brutes." The solution proposed by some US politicians has been to add more humanities courses as study requirements for medical students. But what patients truly want is to be treated with compassion: they want someone to care. This article asks (and attempts to answer) an important question: "Is curiosity the same, in some cases, as caring?" Common wisdom holds that adding humanities studies to medical curricula will make the physician a more complete human being. Dr. Fitzgerald argues instead that "humane people are curious and therefore choose to explore the humanities as well as the sciences." Curious physicians make for better caregivers by spending more time with their patients, demonstrating interest and care. This alone can have some therapeutic effect. Curiosity not only leads physicians to make better diagnoses, it also provides the opportunity to share for meaningful, sacred, and memorable moments with patients. When teaching new doctors, an excellent attending identifies students with an innate curiosity and helps them to develop that skill. Being a curious physician will improve not only the patient's health, but that of the physician as well, and the vitality of the art and science of medicine.

Boissy A, Windover AK, Bokar D, et al. Communication skills training for physicians improves patient satisfaction. J Gen Intern Med 2016;31:755–61.

As a physician, having an aptitude for skillful communication provides a critical path to improved patient satisfaction. This study at the Cleveland Clinic included 1,500 attending physicians who underwent a communication skills training session and nearly 2,000 controls who did not. The eight-hour experiential training session, developed by the Cleveland Clinic Center for Excellence in Healthcare Communication, functioned as the intervention in this study. The study then used common measures of patient satisfaction and physician wellness to determine the impact of the training intervention. While the results showed modest, indirect improvements to patient satisfaction, they also demonstrated stronger improvements to physician empathy while decreasing burnout symptoms (i.e., emotional exhaustion, depersonalization, personal accomplishment). The primary takeaway from these results is that a training program centered on relationship-centered communication skills can improve patient outcomes and significantly improve physician empathy and self-efficacy while reducing symptoms of burnout.

11

The Sacred Act of Healing

*The greatest mistake in the treatment of diseases is that there
are physicians for the body and physicians for the soul, although the two cannot be separated.*

—Plato

As we discussed in a previous chapter, healthcare that champions the
relationship between patient and physician has become a key goal of
the American medical establishment. In its 2001 report "Crossing
the Quality Chasm," the Institute of Medicine issued a call for doctors
to be "respectful of and responsive to individual patient preferences,
needs, and values," and to ensure that "patient values guide all clinical decisions."[1] The patient's experience of the healthcare journey
is an important outcome that is carefully monitored and reported.
As such, the antiquated physician-centric model of hospital care has
been replaced with one in which the patient's values and viewpoints
are not merely metrics to strive toward but foundational to effective care. Indeed, when patients connect with their physician, their
health improves.[2,3]

Such concern for the centrality of the relationship has been touted
before. A century ago, for example, when the eminent physician
Francis W. Peabody was writing his influential essays and books, he
penned the often-quoted, "One of the essential qualities of the clinician is interest in humanity, for the secret of the care of the patient is
in caring for the patient."[4] Dr. Peabody also addressed the common
complaint that the era's medical school graduates (then, mostly

Teaching Inpatient Medicine. Second Edition. Nathan Houchens, Molly Harrod, and Sanjay Saint,
Oxford University Press. © Nathan Houchens, Molly Harrod, and Sanjay Saint 2023.
DOI: 10.1093/oso/9780197639023.003.0011

men) were more engaged with the mechanisms of disease than with
the care of their patients.

> The good physician knows his patients through and through, and his
> knowledge is bought dearly. Time, sympathy, and understanding must
> be lavishly dispensed, but the reward is to be found in that personal
> bond which forms the greatest satisfaction of the practice of medicine.[4]

This dedication to form bonds is a core characteristic for our 18
attending physicians. It is reflected in a comment one of them made
to her team after an interaction with a patient grappling with substance use: "The longer you stay with a patient, the more you will
identify with them, see yourself in them." Another of our exemplary
attendings put forth a statement that might well serve as a message to
medical students everywhere. "The patient's room is a sacred place,"
he said, "and it's a privilege for us to be in there. And if we don't earn
that privilege, then we don't get to go there."

This chapter expands on the previous discussion of communication and shows how our attendings demonstrate care, through their
words and actions, for patients in that sacred place—and how they
serve as role models for their learners in the process. The attendings'
behavior with their patients, how they manifest the very best of the
"hidden curriculum," often establishes the standard that learners
will emulate throughout their professional careers.

A Representative Interaction

Each encounter we witnessed between one of our attendings and a
patient was, of course, a unique occasion, but many of them were
markedly similar to the moments set forth here. As any effective
doctor would, the attending used his interviewing and examination skills effectively to weigh the patient's symptoms and history,
ultimately deciding on a course of action. Through empathy and
humor, he established a positive, collaborative connection with
both the patient's mother and the patient that eased the way for rich

information sharing about the patient's family history. Here is an abbreviated version of what we observed.

The team entered the patient's room, and the attending quickly struck up a conversation with the patient's mother. They spoke about how many children she had and laughingly discussed whether the patient was a "good son" or not. The attending showed us the patient's fingernails, which were hyperpigmented. "You should see how bad my toenails are," the patient said. When the attending wanted to check his feet, the patient resisted. "My own wife hasn't seen my toes for 10 years," he said, but he eventually allowed a peek.

Attending: Those aren't so bad. Do you work somewhere where your feet get wet?

Patient: I'm a cook.

Attending: So water is probably splashing on your feet. That's what happens. Are you lifting things at work?

Patient: I can't do that anymore.

[Additional discussion about work activities performed.]

Attending: [To patient] I was thinking about you last night, and I want the GI [gastrointestinal] people to see you.

The patient's mother asked the attending whether her son had cancer, pointing out that it had struck both sides of his family. During his hospital stay, her son had undergone extensive testing and evaluation without showing any signs of cancer, the attending replied, but he repeated his call for a GI consultation. As the team began to leave the room, the attending stayed back to have a few private words with the patient's mother. We heard him quietly say, "I know you are worried about your boy. We're taking care of him."

Preparation Paves the Way

"I actually used to like going in cold in the morning with no clue about what's coming," one of our attendings told us. Now, like most of the other 18, he reads up on new patients before he meets with his team. Knowing patients' lab values and medical history not only saves time on rounds, it also frees up parts of the mind to focus more intently on patient interactions. With effective preparation, physicians can have a plan prepared which allows them to carefully listen to their patients rather than scramble to remember details of their care. It also means that the up-to-date attendings can, in the words of a current learner, "quickly identify subtle differences in the way patients present and be aware of some of their laboratory abnormalities that may potentially be related to their chief complaint." And it helps attendings plan their mornings more efficiently because they know which patients have more complex problems and will thus require extra time.

The attendings also read up on their patients because of duty hour restrictions. "You have to have a full picture of what's going on with a patient before most of the team," one of the attendings explained. "It's impossible for the single team member left with knowledge of the patients to handle all the questions and calls."

The fact that their attendings are so knowledgeable about their patients can be a spur to learners. "Maybe other attendings might be a little more lax with what happened 10 years ago and wouldn't push us to look as deeply into charts," a current learner said. "Our attending always knows what's going on in-depth, and that pushes all of us to do the same."

Patient Protection Takes Various Forms

In matters large and small, the 18 attendings are aware that they are role models for their learners, and they behave accordingly. As a part of their role modeling, they undertake specific actions that serve to protect their patients. For instance, attendings directly work to protect their patients from infection that can be spread within the hospital. Before and after every patient, they use antiseptic gel or wash their hands with soap and water, depending on the circumstances. They wear gloves when examining patients' wounds. They keep their stethoscopes clean.

The attendings take great care in every aspect of their clinical work, especially to ensure that the right patient receives the right care at the right time. We observed a team dive right into the rhythm of a newly arrived electrocardiogram (EKG), when their attending paused the discussion: "First, make sure it's for this patient. There's nothing worse than going through a whole EKG to find out it wasn't your patient."

Our attendings are thorough and empathic, especially when examining patients. They warm their stethoscopes before use and auscultate directly on the patient's body. "She does it the right way every time," a current learner said of his attending. "You can see other attendings auscultate over gowns or clothing, but you see she's doing it the way it was taught and that's what you want to emulate." This simple action enhances diagnostic accuracy to help the patient even more. During the physical exam, the attendings each have their own individual techniques. "He has a very distinct way," a former learner said of his attending, "deciding which parts are the most important to do to go down the diagnostic algorithm of why this patient has shoulder pain."

As discussed in earlier chapters, many of the 18 attendings are not shy about admitting what they don't know. When they lack a clear diagnosis, would benefit from education by an expert, or are stumped about the appropriate treatment, they will call for a subspecialty consultation to ensure the patient receives the best care. Automatic consultation is not their default position, however. A former learner described his attending: "He takes ownership and responsibility. He is really, 'I know what's going on and I'll consult you [the specialist] when I *really* need you, not just for the sake of it.'"

The attendings want to protect their patients from the various potential threats to them while in the hospital. One way some of them accomplish this is by getting their patients up from bed and walking as soon as possible—for diagnostic reasons and to assess the safety of the patient's movements. "It's better than laboratory tests, fancy CT [computed tomography] scans," a former learner said, echoing his attending. "Walking the patient around the room, pushing the pole, closing the back of the gown so they don't expose themselves to everybody, and making sure the Foley [catheter] is not pulling any-thing. It's not always an easy thing to do, but my attending would do it all the time."

The 18 attendings' focus on the patient's physical condition doesn't end with a firm diagnosis and clinical stability. They seek to continue protecting their patients by constantly looking for new ways to think through the patient's situation, taking nothing for granted. In a sense, they are anticipating trouble: hoping for the best while preparing for the worst. One of the attendings asked his team where their patient with diabetes was injecting himself with insulin. Too many times in the same spot, he warned, and there would be a danger of neurop-athy and of shortening the medicine's half-life. This served to both teach the team and engage the patient in their care.

Connections with Patients at the Bedside

Relationship-centered care can yield significant benefits for both physicians and patients. When physicians and patients feel connected, and when patients become actively engaged in their care, good things can happen. For our attendings, the good things happen at the bedside. "[Talking] outside of the room, going through lab values in front of a computer, you lose the connection with the pa-tient," a current learner said, reflecting his attending's views. "This is a person we are treating. These are her lab values, and this is her life right now. It's everything to her. She should be part of the dis-cussion." Here we expand on points made in a prior chapter about the ways in which our attendings form bonds with patients at their bedsides.

Making First Impressions and Discussing Nonmedical Topics

The 18 attendings cultivate relationships by demonstrating, in dozens of ways, their empathy and respect for every patient. They smile as they enter a patient's room, seeking to set a positive and friendly tone for the encounter. They introduce themselves and their team members to the patient if it's a first visit. Attendings quickly size up the situation of the patient, looking to her comfort. "Is the sunlight bothering your eyes?" one of the attendings asked a patient and proceeded to close the window blinds. Another recognized and normalized the inherent frustration that can bubble up when a medical team interrupts a meal in the hospital by saying to the patient, "I don't like it when people roll up when I'm eating." And, at the end of the conversation: "Thank you for letting us interrupt your grits." Our attendings will usually find a way to create a pleasant verbal exchange with the patient, tailoring their approach to the individual.

"All right, rock star," an attending said to a patient. "Tell me the story behind all those bracelets you're wearing." Laughing, the patient showed the attending his favorite. The attending read it aloud, "Don't be stupid," and added, "Words we can all live by."

One of our attendings has traveled widely in the United States, and he often starts conversations with patients by asking where they come from because, chances are, he's been there and can connect through discussions about the place. He's also served in the military, so his opening gambit with veterans is, "What branch of the service were you in?" Attendings may ask the names and types of pets. They may ask about the most memorable or proudest moment in the patient's life. An attending told us, "I just show patients I'm interested in them as people, and you can see the effect it has. It's part of being a good doctor."

It is worth highlighting that the behaviors our attendings use to form connections with patients mirrors those same behaviors they use to form connections with their learners.

Responding to Physical and Emotional Needs

Attendings' empathy becomes particularly evident when the patient is in pain or distress. In one instance, an attending stayed by the patient's side, stroking her arm, telling her to breathe slowly, while requesting more pain medication. "I'm sorry you're in so much pain," the attending said several times. When leaving, the attending asked one of the team members to stay with the patient until the new medication was administered.

During our interviews, we talked with a current learner about his attending as role model and the special relationship his attending creates with his patients. "My experience is that patients don't really know whether they're being treated appropriately," the learner said. "They don't know that this medication is better than that medication for such and such a reason. My attending actually is just the best at managing patients medically. But he has also gone beyond the traditional scope of a physician in the sense that he is meeting patients' emotional needs—and that's pretty rare. It's something I'm really hoping to take with me."

Engaging Patients Through Analogies and Teach-Back

During the physical examination, attendings seek to make sure the process is as free from discomfort and embarrassment as possible. Their exam technique is thorough, yet gentle and informative. One attending prepared each patient for the examination by saying, "I'm going to tell you everything I'm about to do before I do it." We listened in on another at the bedside who described the examination technique and what it shows using an analogy that most people can appreciate: "A few of us are going to listen to you this morning. I'm going on the other side, so you'll have one of us on each side of you. . . . Can you turn your head? We want to look at your neck. This is like a gas gauge and will let us know if you are full or empty of fluid." Curtains are drawn around the bed for privacy, and gowns are closed back up when the exam is over. The attendings will often use a comforting touch, particularly at the end of the exam. A hand on the patient's hand or shoulder is but another way to signal connection.

As part of their dedication to patient-centeredness, our attendings keep their patients in the loop. After the physical exam, for instance, the attendings would tell a patient that they were going to "talk shop" with their team to discuss their findings but would translate what was said into lay language after the jargon-laden discussion. To make sure their patients understood their diagnosis and treatment plan, the attendings would regularly engage in "teach-back" methods. They would ask patients, "Tell me what we're up to," or, "Tell me what our plan is." Some have suggested to put the onus of effective explanation back on the physician[5] by saying something like, "To make sure I did a good job explaining, could you let me know what you are taking away from this conversation?" Others still will bring family members and loved ones into the process: "When you talk with your sister about this conversation, what will you tell her?"

In the following exchange, one of our attendings explained to a patient and his wife the procedure being considered to prevent blood clots from going from his legs to his lungs.

Attending: Do you play badminton?

Wife: I have.

Attending: So have I, and I bet I could beat you [he says jokingly]. But you know the little birdie? Well, this procedure we're thinking about, there's a net that looks like the birdie and it would be inside him and it's used to catch all the blood clots. Doing that would keep a situation like this [pulmonary embolism] from happening again, and he would feel better. He does have to be on Coumadin the rest of his life, so no more mixed martial arts fighting or throwing plates at his head.

[Conversation continued with the attending asking about another family member who was also diagnosed with the same clotting disorder. The attending recommended they discuss it with their children's pediatrician, since the disorder could be hereditary.]

In addition to demonstrating the attending's desire to keep his patients informed as clearly as possible, the preceding exchange illustrates other elements of his relationship-centered approach, including his use of humor and his concern for the patient's family. In fact, the 18 attendings are fully committed to keeping their patients' families up to date on patients' condition and prognosis. "He's always having a family meeting or calling a patient's wife to tell her what we did today and the plan," a former learner recalled of his attending. Our attendings are also in touch with their patients' ambulatory clinic physicians, alerting them to their patients' presence in the hospital and keeping them aware of major developments.

Getting at Eye Level and Exploring the Patient's Lived Experience

When they talk with their patients, the attendings often kneel down or sit on a stool in order to talk eye to eye (see Figure 11.1). "I feel you're able to connect with people much better that way than if you're towering over them," one of the attendings said. She went on: "It's a horrible power dynamic to be sick and someone's standing over you telling you things."

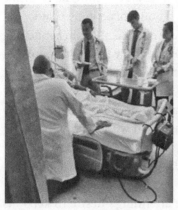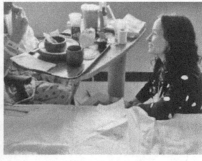

Figure 11.1 Attendings kneeling at patients' bedsides.

Another attending told us that kneeling by the bedside sends patients a message: "You think it's uncomfortable? Damn right! It hurts." The point of the message? "It's just to remind them, we don't lord over the patient," he said. "This is their place."

During their talks with patients, the attendings speak calmly and slowly. And they listen, patiently and carefully. A former learner described his attending "sitting through everything the patients said, even when they were saying a million things that didn't really make a whole lot of sense."

Physicians can learn a great deal from listening to their patients. They learn about aspects of the patients' and their families' medical history that can shed light on current conditions and treatments. Physicians can also get a line on patients' personalities, which can help form a stronger bond. Here's how one of our attendings applied that knowledge in working with a patient who had just undergone open heart surgery but was declining to take pain medications: "Someone took a saw to your breastbone! [It's okay] if you need pain meds. And it will make it a lot easier for you to do your rehabilitation." Thereafter, the patient decided to try some medication.

Knowledge of the details of patients' lives can also be invaluable in planning for their departure from the hospital and resumption of their outpatient lives. "We have a patient who is very sick," a current learner told us, "and our attending learned that the patient's wife was admitted at another institution in the same city. Right away, he realized that was going to be a problem when the patient went home. Who would take care of him? So, we had our social worker and case manager talk with [the other institution's social worker] to work out a solution."

Our attendings start thinking about their patients' hospital discharge as soon as they are admitted to the hospital. A current learner described her attending's early outpatient focus: "It seems like she always has a plan, like, 'Oh, by the way, when this patient leaves, they're going to need this, this, and this. You should start on that now.'"

The attendings' outpatient focus extended beyond medical care to encompass the financial needs of their patients. We heard an attending talking to her team: "What was the purpose of our palliative care conversation yesterday? To consider the patient's insurance.

She has Medicaid that might affect the amount of palliative care [she is eligible for]."

Departing the Sacred Place

The final stage of a team's encounter receives careful attention from the 18 attendings. Following the physical examination, one attending remarked to her team "Okay, let's get her back up in bed, so she's more comfortable." As another attending said, "You make sure the room is how you left it when you walked in. You turn off the lights if they were off; you take care of the bedrails; you fix the TV volume." One attending specifically called this act of kindness out: "Were you watching that movie? We'll put it back on for you." They also offer patients a pleasant, upbeat farewell along the lines of "It's a pleasure meeting you," "Good to see you," or "It's a beautiful day."

The next chapter acknowledges the inherent challenges to the patient–provider relationship presented by the COVID-19 pandemic and other crises. While many relationship-centered communication practices (such as physical touch and kneeling to the patient's level) needed to stop during this time, we learn from local experience and research the ways that attendings navigated these challenges and continued to lead by example.

Main Points

1. Attendings treat their patients with respect, empathy, and dignity. Even though their encounters might be brief, attendings make it a priority to get to know their patients and build rapport. Developing and cultivating these relationships helps the team plan for the patient's care within and outside of the hospital.

2. Attendings spend time explaining to patients, in lay language and with analogies, what they are thinking and how they are

approaching the patient's treatment. They often sit down or kneel when speaking to patients so they can be on the same level.

3. Attendings keep in mind their patients' lives outside the hospital, planning early for discharge and demonstrating concern over their social and financial needs.

Further Reading

Collier KM, James CA, Saint S, Howell JD. Is it time to more fully address teaching religion and spirituality in medicine? Ann Intern Med 2020;172:817–8.

This Ideas and Opinions article from *Annals of Internal Medicine* provides a brief history of the view of spirituality and religion in medicine and addresses patients' desires to incorporate faith into their care. The authors argue that as the scientific model took shape and faith fell outside of it, little room has been reserved for things that cannot be scientifically measured. Learner "comfort with ambiguity" is a benchmark in numerous association recommendations and teaching guidelines. However, students learn from example in watching their instructors discuss (or not discuss) a spiritual history. The authors parallel taking a spiritual history to the previously "taboo" subject of sexual history and urge discussion of patients' beliefs to provide patient-centered care.

Mullan F. A founder of quality assessment encounters a troubled system firsthand. Health Aff 2001;20:137–41.

In this article, Avedis Donabedian, a physician, scholar, and poet, is interviewed by Fitzhugh Mullan shortly before his death. The topics covered included Donabedian's reflections on being a patient, his personal feeling on the quality of care he had received, and his sense of confidence in the day-to-day management of his care. In response to a question regarding his feelings about the rapid commercialization of healthcare in recent years, Donabedian responded, "Ultimately, the secret quality is love. You have to love your patient, you have to love your profession, you have to love your God. If you have love, you can then work backward to monitor and improve the system."

Peabody FW. The care of the patient. JAMA 1927;88:877–82.

In this essay, Peabody stresses that one simply cannot become a skillful practitioner of medicine in the time allotted for training in medical school. He emphasizes that medicine is not a trade to be learned but rather a profession to be entered; it is a profession that requires continuous study and prolonged experience taking care of patients. Peabody addresses three main topics: the importance of individualizing medical care, a call for awareness that hospitalization can be a dehumanizing experience, and the care of patients whose cause of symptoms cannot be diagnosed.

Hartzband P, Groopman J. Keeping the patient in the equation: Humanism and health care reform. N Engl J Med 2009;361:554–5.

In this article, the authors discuss two movements that have emerged in recent decades: medical humanism and evidence-based practice. Although both movements aim to improve patient care, their approaches to accomplishing this goal differ. Humanism aims to understand the patient as a person, focusing on individual values, goals, and preferences, whereas evidence-based practice aims to put medicine on a firmer scientific footing using data and clinical guidance to standardize procedures and therapies. They point out the obstacles these two movements may face, as well as how they may coalesce rather than conflict with one another.

12

Caring During Crisis

A crisis is an opportunity riding a dangerous wind.

—Chinese proverb

In March 2020, the first patient in the United States was diagnosed with severe acute respiratory syndrome coronavirus-2 (SARS-CoV-2), better known as COVID-19. This novel viral pandemic has become the greatest global public health crisis in this century. Since that time, the foundation of healthcare—truly the entire world—has undergone seismic transformations due to the immense strain placed on individuals and healthcare systems to accommodate the tremendous influx of patients seeking care.

Healthcare leaders, administrators, clinicians, facilities experts, logistics, infection prevention, and countless other groups coordinated and aligned their goals of rapid expansion to care for as many patients as possible as safely as possible. New inpatient units were constructed; precious resources including personal protective equipment (PPE) and mechanical ventilators were deployed and frequently rationed to those patients who needed them the most; healthcare employees volunteered or were reassigned to work in different units; and they received new information on care protocols—sometimes as frequently as every hour. These rapidly changing circumstances, knowledge, and processes required immense flexibility, adaptability, and incorporation of constant change from everyone. And this, of course, included teaching attending physicians.

A brief disclaimer: None of our research team's observations or interviews of the 18 exemplary attending physicians was conducted

Teaching Inpatient Medicine. Second Edition. Nathan Houchens, Molly Harrod, and Sanjay Saint,
Oxford University Press. © Nathan Houchens, Molly Harrod, and Sanjay Saint 2023.
DOI: 10.1093/oso/9780197639023.003.0012

during the COVID-19 pandemic nor during any other known natural crises. Previously discussed observations, anecdotes, and examples of teaching approaches did *not* reflect the mammoth changes required by all during the pandemic. The reader should recognize that many of the aforementioned techniques and behaviors needed to be adjusted to mitigate the risk of transmission from this deadly viral pathogen. Thus, we cannot draw from our 18 attendings for this chapter. Rather, we rely on local experiences and strategies by teaching attendings and healthcare system leaders to lead by example in providing etiquette-based medicine and shift the focus from guiding effective teaching as the main priority to existential and logistical support for patients and learners.

In 2008, Michael Khan described six core principles of etiquette-based medicine to consider in order to demonstrate care while interacting with patients.[1] Throughout prior chapters of this book, the reader has seen countless examples of exemplary attendings employing etiquette-based medicine and role-modeling these behaviors for their team members. How then did these behaviors continue or change as a result of the COVID-19 pandemic? Our local attendings recognized that the same core philosophies and principles applied and were in fact even more crucial because of the inherent uncertainty, unease, and apprehension most patients experienced when hospitalized with COVID-19 or with other conditions during surges of the COVID-19 pandemic. They once again led by example.

Asking permission (for instance, "Is now an okay time to talk?") prior to entering the room of a hospitalized patient is a sign of respect. Even though patients were being interviewed virtually in their hospital rooms, attendings continued to begin the conversation this way. And because of restrictions on visitors entering the hospital wards, more and more update conversations with patients' loved ones were held via telephone call or virtual video conference. It was again a sign of respect and empathy to ask permission—and importantly, to avoid assuming the person on the other end is constantly available and ready to discuss updates—before delving into important conversations.

Hospitalized patients are often seen by multiple members of the healthcare team, including physicians, nursing staff, physical therapists, social workers, technicians, and dietitians, to name but a few. We found it helpful to introduce members of the team, particularly since facemasks and other forms of personal protective equipment (PPE) were in use during the COVID-19 pandemic. It is entirely conceivable, even highly likely, that a patient would never see the full faces of the individuals caring for them; indeed, some team members never saw each other's faces. To mitigate this, our local medicine service created team "facesheets" that included a brief paragraph recognizing how hard it is to be in the hospital during these uncertain times, along with photographs, names, and roles of each team member (see Figure 12.1). This small but impactful intervention was seen as a way to better forge connections between patient and providers.

In order to avoid COVID-19 transmission, handshakes— previously a cornerstone of many cultures' greetings and closings— needed to be replaced with other expressions of respect. Seeing the value, attendings substituted with a wave, a bow, or a Namaste salutation. And since patients and families have a difficult time reading facial and emotional cues when the provider is wearing a facemask,[2] smiles were often supplemented with verbal statements of kindness.

The value of getting at eye level and showing that the patient has the attending's full attention has been described in the medical literature and cannot be overstated.[3] Patients feel more comfortable and even perceive that their doctors spend more time with them if they sit compared with when they stand (even when the actual time spent is the same). Many hospitals, including ours, have folding chairs or seats on which physicians and other healthcare team members can sit to ensure this important act continues without increasing the risk of microbial transmission.

Once again, the technique of explaining one's role on the team was challenged by the need for PPE, such as gowns that covered white coats and masks that obscured facial features. The facesheet example above helped patients feel more at ease with members of their team and better recall the roles they played on the team. We witnessed

Dear Veteran –

These are scary times for all. We want you to know you are in the hands of those who care about your health. It can be hard to feel connected when you cannot see a person's face, so we thought you might want to see what we look like when we are not wearing masks and other equipment:

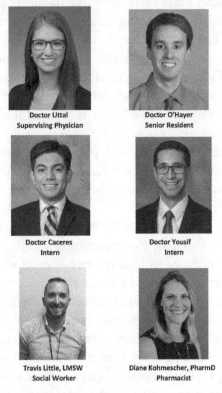

Doctor Uttal
Supervising Physician

Doctor O'Hayer
Senior Resident

Doctor Caceres
Intern

Doctor Yousif
Intern

Travis Little, LMSW
Social Worker

Diane Kohmescher, PharmD
Pharmacist

Thank you for your service to our country. It is now our honor to serve you.

Thank you for choosing the VA Ann Arbor!

Emerald Medicine Team

Figure 12.1 Team "facesheet" displaying team members' names and roles provided to patients.

local attendings reintroducing themselves and reorienting patients to their roles on a daily basis rather than just on the first meeting.

Just as they did before the pandemic, attendings continued to ask their patients how they were feeling about being in the hospital. However, within the context of COVID-19, attendings approached these conversations with a new recognition that, for many patients, the hospital had become an even more frightening, foreign, and isolating place. Responding to apprehension, fear, anxiety, and frustration with empathy became even more important to build the partnership between patient and physician.

The simple acts of physical distancing and wearing PPE created multiple challenges to achieving effective communication. During face-to-face conversations, actual physical barriers such as distance and facemasks imposed new hindrances on all types of communication.[4] A technique our attendings used was the incorporation of clear facemasks. These allowed better patient recognition of expressions, empathic responses, and visual facial cues from the physician. Attendings inquired with patients about sensory disturbances and thereafter arranged for assistive devices to enhance their senses of sight and sound. Attendings articulated, increased the volume of their speech, and clearly enunciated their words to overcome the barrier created by the facemask. Communication with families and caregivers needed to occur much more frequently over the telephone or via video calls due to visitor restrictions. For many, this created a sense of impersonality, which needed to be addressed through empathetic statements.

During times of crisis, it is clear that an important part of the teaching attending's role is to model effective communication with patients and families. What becomes more apparent, also, is that these skills often mirror those used when interacting with their own team members. Many attendings noticed a shift in their focus from educational guides to sources of support. The worry, apprehension, and frustration patients and families were feeling were the same emotions expressed, either explicitly or implicitly, by learners and other members of the healthcare team. And so attendings used the same principles and approaches with their team.

On an existential level, attendings emphasized the importance of personal health, self-care, and the safety and well-being of the learner's family members. Attendings acknowledged the emotions that were likely under the surface and demonstrated humility and partnership. Learners were not alone, they said: everyone was grappling together. It was clear that teaching attendings were no longer the heads of teams but rather positioned themselves alongside learners and regularly showed their own vulnerability. Attendings often discussed reignited hobbies or new activities that the learners had recently been taken up. This was one way that attendings engaged their team in discussions of how they are staying healthy—physically, mentally, emotionally, and spiritually.

On a more logistical level, attendings and health system leaders supported learners with the core elements of Maslow's hierarchy of needs. They ensured that the physical team space available to learners was amenable to work without putting the team at risk of potential COVID-19 transmission. Attendings and health system leaders often worked to provide learners with regular lunches to both recognize and appreciate their efforts and allow them one less stressor with which to deal. Attendings and leaders provided appropriate PPE and encouraged personal safety to avoid illness—and when illness did strike, they were quick to encourage rest and recovery until the learner felt comfortable to return or the requisite amount of time had passed. In recognition of the fact that more frequent check-ins with family members often led to more responsibilities than before the pandemic, teaching attendings rolled up their sleeves and took on these less traditional attending roles by putting in orders, writing notes, contacting family members, and coordinating care with outpatient providers. In all these ways, exemplary attendings demonstrated support for their learners to alleviate some of the immense stress and strain they were under.

Up to this point in the book, we have reported our observations and interview details of the 18 outstanding attending physicians and others, trusting that our readers would be drawn to follow their eminent footsteps. In the next and final chapter, we take a different tack. We will recast our most important findings as recommendations. We hope that readers will find this more direct and simplified form valuable in the evolution of their own careers as attendings.

Main Points

1. Intentional, alternative actions were taken to respectfully communicate with patients, despite distancing and decreased face-to-face interaction from COVID protocols. Healthcare providers acknowledged the unique difficulties of being a patient during this time.
2. Attendings positioned themselves alongside learners rather than at the head of the team. They did so by showing vulnerability and acknowledging fears and concerns, instilling a true "team" mentality.
3. Attendings sometimes took on tasks outside of their traditional role in order to show support of learners and reduce stress levels of those on the team.

Further Reading

Houchens N, Tipirneni R. Compassionate communication amid the COVID-19 pandemic. J Hosp Med 2020;15:437–9.

    In this perspective from June 2020, the authors address challenges that arose from communication barriers during COVID-19, as well as opportunities to overcome them by connecting with patients to deliver high-quality care. The authors present a concise summary of three groups to focus on to ensure compassionate communication: patients, families and caregivers, and the healthcare team. For each group, the authors identify four to five strategies that can help overcome barriers to be able to continue providing compassionate care despite the limitations imposed to protect everyone during the COVID-19 pandemic.

Arora VM, Chivu M, Schram A, Meltzer D. Implementing physical distancing in the hospital: A key strategy to prevent nosocomial transmission of COVID-19. J Hosp Med 2020;15:290–1.

    This very early look from April 2020 into COVID-19 prevention measures examines a concept everyone is now familiar with: physical distancing. Although a relatively foreign concept to many before COVID-19 swept across the world, the authors emphasize this simple strategy to reduce transmission of the virus in the hospital by providing specific strategies based on those implemented at the University of Chicago medical center. These included many of the essential components of physical distancing: make meetings, rounding, and sign-out virtual, and give people in the hospital space to work safely at computers and to have call room space.

Edigin E, Eseaton PO, Shaka H, Ojemolon PE, Asemota IR, Akuna E. Impact of COVID-19 pandemic on medical postgraduate training in the United States. Med Educ Online 2020;25:1774318.

Providing an early look into the impact COVID-19 had on medical training, this June 2020 perspective discusses the immediate educational and healthcare impacts of the pandemic. The Association of American Medical Colleges (AAMC) decided that, if continuing in their traditional roles, it would not be possible to keep all medical students safe, so they were removed from their clinical clerkships, while residents and fellows continued to perform clinical work. As outpatient visits transitioned to virtual care models (using telephone and video calls), the volume of patients and diversity of disease processes seen dropped appreciably. Similarly, delaying care for non–life-threatening health conditions for people who would otherwise have ended up as inpatients on hospital services reduced the opportunities for medical learners to practice many skills. Additionally, many organizations used trainees to bolster aspects of their COVID-19 response. The cancelation of research conferences, questions about travel for international medical graduates who had been accepted to US residency programs that year, and disruptions to the postgraduate recruitment process were all concerns as the country and world dealt with a completely strange world that was adapting to COVID.

Fihn SD. COVID-19: Back to the future. JAMA Intern Med 2020;180:1149–50.

This perspective from July 2020 examines the many disruptions to "normal" care caused by COVID-19 surging through an unprepared healthcare system in the United States. From repurposing specialist hospital space to care for patients with COVID-19 to changes in daily operational leadership, this piece provides an at once urgent and yet hopeful view of the positive effects this pandemic has had in the healthcare world.

13

Putting It All Together

The desire to reach for the stars is ambitious. The desire to reach hearts is wise.

—Maya Angelou

Attending physicians have always borne a weighty responsibility. They take accountability for the quality of their learners' clinical skills and knowledge and, thus, for the level of medical care received by each succeeding generation of patients. They confront myriad challenges, including less time with their teams as a result of limits on learners' work hours, shrinking time with their patients as a result of shorter hospital stays, large interdisciplinary teams of healthcare specialists, increased administrative and documentation requirements, high rates of burnout, increasingly recognized social inequities, an ever-expanding knowledge base, healthcare crises like the COVID-19 pandemic, and a sicker, more complex patient population. Yet, despite these challenges, these attending physicians continue to inspire new generations and approach their craft as bastions of wisdom and compassion.

We intended our study of 18 of these outstanding attending physicians to capture their respective "lightning in a bottle" to help today's attendings manage these remarkable circumstances. We believed that a detailed, multiperspective description of the instructional, clinical, and humanistic methods of these remarkable attendings would yield a trove of practical, actionable advice for internal medicine physicians and physicians-in-training.

Teaching Inpatient Medicine. Second Edition. Nathan Houchens, Molly Harrod, and Sanjay Saint, Oxford University Press. © Nathan Houchens, Molly Harrod, and Sanjay Saint 2023. DOI: 10.1093/oso/9780197639023.003.0013

In this final chapter, we recap that advice, encompassing many of the 18 attendings' most important strategies, attitudes, and practices.

A Safe, Supportive Learning Environment

High-quality clinical education is collaborative rather than authoritative—cooperative rather than competitive. Learners are more comfortable and reach higher achievements when there are diverse perspectives and the learning environment is safe, welcoming, and supportive rather than anxiety-provoking and demeaning. Teaching attendings can create this kind of environment in the following ways.

Establish Personal Connections and Build Trust

Address team members with respect, call them by their first names, and get to know them as people. If team members are comfortable with you personally, they will feel safe and comfortable on rounds. Whenever possible, target teaching points to the individual learner's interests. Establish high but achievable expectations and push learners with positivity. Allow learners autonomy to make patient care decisions while also ensuring appropriate support and supervision.

Appreciate Diversity

Individuals from historically marginalized or minoritized groups face many challenges simply because of their identities. These challenges include discrimination, unconscious bias, and harassment, to name a few. Many also grapple with imposter syndrome. Recognize these challenges because of their prevalence and their negative effects on individuals in healthcare. Work to understand the various strategies that women, underrepresented minorities in medicine, and other groups may use to navigate these issues while supporting one another with compassion, understanding, and grace.

Be a Learner

Position yourself as a *member* of the team rather than the *leader* of the team. Show your team members that, as a coach, you are a lifelong learner just like them. Be available (sometimes this means postponing other responsibilities) and eager to help team members and learn with them. Engage in self-discipline, monitor your progress, and always strive to improve your own clinical and teaching skills. William Osler said, "Medicine is a science of uncertainty and an art of probability." For those who feel they can, consider admitting when you are wrong, when you do not know, and demonstrating humility by sharing your own medical errors and gaps in knowledge.

Exude Warmth and Enthusiasm

Create a warm, welcoming, and accepting environment through your communication. Avoid interrupting learners' presentations, give praise liberally, and be approachable. Epitomize the positive aspects of the hidden curriculum through respectful collaboration with all members of the healthcare team. Set an example by outwardly showing your pleasure in caring for patients and improving the environment. Use humor, a smile, and a vested interest in people to show you care.

Keep Interactions and Feedback Positive

Explore potential mistakes first rather than making accusations, and reframe mistakes into learning opportunities. Use improvisational skills like saying "yes, and . . ." to build on learners' suggestions and show support while gently redirecting or guiding the conversation and their thought processes. Honesty without kindness is cruelty: feedback is an inevitable part of the attending's role, but it is important to provide modifying feedback with kindness (and, if significant, in private) and remember that you were once a learner also.

Lead and Mentor

Recognize the impact that leadership has on team outcomes and the roles mentors and sponsors play for guiding physicians in their careers. When mentoring others, work to avoid gender scripts and archetypes, promote reciprocal learning, and be the change you want to see by supporting mentees who may have different amounts of social capital. Consider your role as a traditional mentor, coach, sponsor, or connector, and note that the specific role often depends on the mentee's stated needs and goals. Apply mindfulness when mentoring others to positively impact the relationship. To mentor individuals in younger generations, try to embrace innovation, purpose, autonomy, and networking while avoiding inertia, busywork, isolation, and strict hierarchies.

Teaching on Rounds

Given time limitations and other responsibilities, exemplary attendings carefully prepare for and maximize every moment with the team. They select and adapt a particular rounding style, engage all team members, and use questions to both assess for learner understanding of concepts and foster the key skill of clinical reasoning. They do all this while remaining flexible so that they may roll with the inevitable unexpected challenges.

Consider Rounding Style and Structure

Tailor your teaching to key time periods during the day to maximize team efficiency—this often takes the form of facilitating short pearls of wisdom rather than long discourses. One rule of thumb: provide a single teaching point per patient per day. Use every opportunity to teach while with the team, even when walking between patient rooms. Consider different formats of oral patient presentations that resonate most with learners' thought processes. Be flexible with rounding style and structure since interruptions and distractions are bound to occur.

Ask Effective Questions Effectively

Engage all team members by targeting questions to every learning level. Pose questions to probe for understanding and to keep learners on their learning edge—this often takes the form of a modest degree of anxiety, an important state to achieve peak performance. All types of questions can be effective, and open-ended questions that prompt learners to explain their thought processes, step by step, are particularly helpful. Avoid lectures filled with facts and factoids. Use "what-if" hypothetical questions to prompt learners to anticipate and prepare for all possible outcomes. Incorporate Socratic questioning—a series of linked questions with each successive question built on the previous answer—to create mental linkages and help learners achieve a richer level of understanding. Avoid the temptation to simply give the answers to questions with which learners are grappling.

Foster and Role Model Clinical Reasoning

Verbalize and make explicit your own rationale for decisions so that learners can understand the thinking of physicians with more experience and different perspectives. Explicitly encourage the use of frameworks for patient conditions to simplify and obviate the need for learners to memorize facts and figures. Encourage critical analysis and questioning of conclusions for both patient care decisions and when interpreting the scholarly literature.

Expand the Team

Include all members of the healthcare team in discussions, give them full respect, and seek their insights and direction in patients' care plans. Nurses, pharmacists, social workers, dieticians, physical therapists, and many others can provide specialized knowledge and unique input for patients. Demonstrate the value that these professionals bring to patient care by referring to them by name and emphasizing their importance to learners and patients.

Adapt to the Unexpected

Healthcare crises such as the COVID-19 pandemic necessitate rapid adjustments in usual activities. During these moments, consider intentional, alternative actions to respectfully communicate with patients and form connections despite literal and metaphorical barriers. Openly acknowledge with patients the unique difficulties of being a patient during these times. Instill a true team mentality by showing your own vulnerability and acknowledging fears and concerns with your team members. Consider taking on tasks outside of your traditional role to show support for learners and reduce their stress levels.

Patient-Centered Learning

The most important teaching takes place at the patient's bedside. The attending is the team's role model and sets the standards for safe and effective patient care. Outstanding teaching attendings recognize that the care of patients is a sacred privilege and that all teaching and learning occurs in the context of the patient. Attendings role-model safety and compassion by washing their hands, listening with the stethoscope on skin instead of over the gown, and putting the patient's socks back on after the examination. They also role-model connection with patients at the bedside through a variety of communication strategies, delineated below.

Teach in the Context of the Patient

Prepare for rounds by reading about each patient and anticipating learner sticking points, teaching topics, and relevant literature before meeting with the team. Always provide instruction in the context of the patient at the bedside so that learners can use this information for subsequent patients. Lessons learned at the bedside are well remembered. Be fully present, detailed, and holistic with the bedside history and examination, both to optimize patient care and to role-model important clinical skills. Role-model coping strategies for the team during challenging moments like unexpected outcomes.

Facilitate Relationship-Centered Communication

Make good use of fundamental communication skills (opening, interviewing and examination, and closing skills) to form connections with patients. Through your words, actions, and empathy, build rapport with patients and their family members, inquire about the patient and their perspectives, and make space for sacred moments to occur. Talk about nonmedical topics in order to connect and relate to the patient's experience and expertise. Talk to patients using layperson language and analogies and assess for understanding by harnessing the "teach-back" technique. Consider your own bodily posture and mannerisms, therapeutic touch, and clothing as important forms of nonverbal communication. Sit down or kneel when speaking to patients so that you are both at eye level.

Plan for the Patient's Future

When patients first arrive, encourage the team to start thinking about their departure from the hospital. Keep in mind patients' lives outside the hospital. Inquire about their social situation, insurance status, and financial needs. How will they get from the hospital to home? Is there anyone at home who can take care of them? Should a team member stay in touch with the patient by telephone? Teach team members to treat all patients as if they were family members.

A Closing Thought

Clinical educators fulfill an important role in the healthcare system. To be an exemplary teaching attending means not only sharing medical knowledge and insights, but also role-modeling what it means to be a compassionate physician in today's healthcare environment. Thus, we leave you with a quote from one of the 18 that represents how the attendings in this study viewed their role as both doctor and teacher: "I think [learners] have to know that you love being a teacher—without declaring it. It has to be obvious. They have to know you care about the craft—the craft of being a doctor."

Further Reading

Wiese J. Teaching in the Hospital. Philadelphia, PA: ACP Press; 2010.

In this useful book edited by one of our 18 attendings, the authors provide hospital-based educators with the tools and techniques needed to be successful in facilitating effective clinical education. Each chapter focuses on a different aspect of teaching and provides examples on such topics as how to establish and communicate expectations and responsibilities; how to conduct rounds in a way that ensures that education complements patient care; how to enhance learning by using illustrations, analogies, mnemonics, and other tricks of the trade; and how to coach learners in the science of clinical reasoning. Clinical problem-based teaching scripts are also provided.

Ludmerer KM. Let Me Heal: The Opportunity to Preserve Excellence in American Medicine. New York, NY: Oxford University Press; 2014.

The author, physician, and historian Kenneth Ludmerer provides an encompassing history of graduate medical education in the United States from its inception to the current day. The author demonstrates how it has changed in response to internal as well as external forces. Ludmerer calls on those within the profession to seize opportunities to improve medical education and thus patient care.

Chopra V, Saint S. "The tunnel at the end of the light": Preparing to attend on the inpatient medical wards. JAMA 2017;318:1007–8.

The transition from other work-related activities and responsibilities to attending on the inpatient medical ward can be very stressful for many. This perspective piece published in *JAMA* offers six helpful tips to help smooth the transition to and from the wards. While these may seem simplistic on the surface, they provide a roadmap to follow to address most of the spaces of the physician's life. Tip 1: Plan ahead for (and around) clinical activities so that you can project out your workload while keeping a careful eye on deadlines. It's important not to forget those you love—maximize quality time with them before service. Tip 2: Prune meetings unrelated to clinical activities. Schedule them after 3 PM if necessary. Tip 3: Set and communicate realistic expectations about your availability when on service. Tip 4: Develop email hygiene by using out-of-office replies to let people know you are on service and by triaging what does not need immediate attention to a special "Service" folder. Tip 5: Finish what can be finished before going on service—especially those items that can be worked on by others while you are on service. Tip 6: Finally, recover: allocate at least half of one day a week during the first few weeks to catch up when you return from service. These modest changes may change your mindset and experience during service.

The 18 Attendings

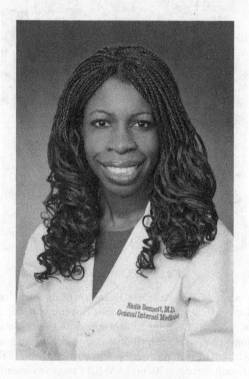

Nadia Bennett, MD, MSEd

Nadia Bennett, MD, MSEd, is Associate Professor of Clinical Medicine at the Hospital of the University of Pennsylvania and Penn Presbyterian Medical Center, and she is Associate Dean of Clinical and Health Systems Sciences Curriculum at the Perelman School of Medicine. She has won numerous teaching awards, including the Provost's Award for Teaching Excellence, Blockley-Osler Award for Excellence in Teaching, and the John M. Eisenberg Teaching Award; she is an Inductee of the Perelman School of Medicine Minority Hall of Fame.

Dr. Bennett received her medical degree from the University of Maryland School of Medicine and completed her internal medicine residency at Duke University Medical Center. She also received her master's degree in Medical Education from the University of Pennsylvania.

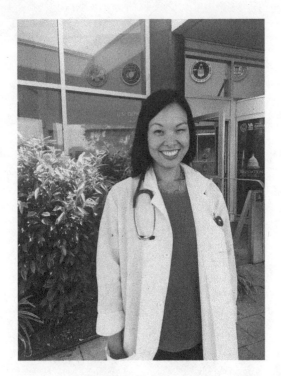

Katherine Chretien, MD

Katherine Chretien, MD, is Associate Dean for Medical Student Affairs and Director of Medical Student Wellness at Johns Hopkins Hospital. She has previously served as Associate Dean for Student Affairs and Professor of Medicine at George Washington University School of Medicine and Health Sciences. She has served as President of Clerkship Directors in Internal Medicine (CDIM) and is on the Northeast Group of Student Affairs (AAMC) Executive Committee. She is the recipient of the Charles H. Griffith III Educational Research Award from CDIM and the Women Leaders in Medicine Award from the American Medical Students Association. She is the editor of the book *Mothers in Medicine: Career, Practice, and Life Lessons Learned* and has also authored the book *I Wish I Read This Book Before Medical School.*

Dr. Chretien received her medical degree from Johns Hopkins University School of Medicine where she also completed the Osler Medical Residency.

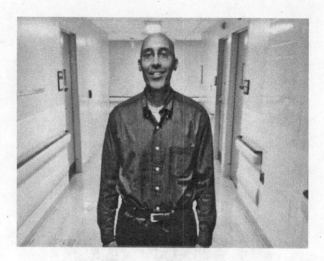

Gurpreet Dhaliwal, MD

Gurpreet Dhaliwal, MD, is a clinician-educator and Professor of Medicine at the University of California at San Francisco (UCSF). He is the site director of the internal medicine clerkships at the San Francisco VA Medical Center, where he teaches medical students and residents in the emergency department, urgent care clinic, inpatient wards, outpatient clinic, and morning report. He has received numerous teaching awards including the Kaiser Award for Teaching Excellence at UCSF and the national Alpha Omega Alpha Robert J. Glaser Distinguished Teaching Award. Dr. Dhaliwal was profiled in a 2012 *New York Times* article as "one of the most skillful clinical diagnosticians in practice today."

Dr. Dhaliwal attended Northwestern University Medical School and was a resident and chief medical resident at UCSF.

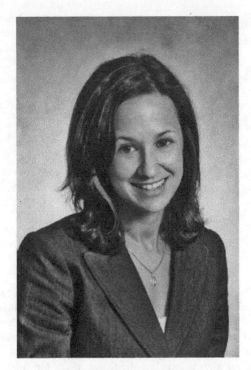

Jeanne Farnan, MD, MHPE

Jeanne M. Farnan, MD, MHPE, is Professor of Medicine, Associate Dean for Medical School Education, and Director of Clinical Skills Education at the University of Chicago Pritzker School of Medicine. Clinically, Dr. Farnan practices as an academic hospitalist and works with Internal Medicine house-staff. She has received the Pre-Clinical Teacher of the Year Award and the Distinguished Educator and Mentor Award at the University of Chicago, and she has written extensively on medical professionalism and education.

Dr. Farnan received her medical degree from the University of Chicago Pritzker School of Medicine and was a resident at the University of Chicago. She received her master's degree in Health Professions Education from the University of Illinois, Chicago.

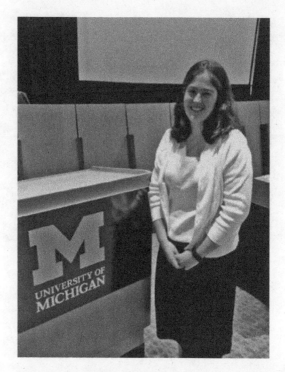

Sarah Hartley, MD, MHPE

Sarah Hartley, MD, MHPE, is Associate Director of the Internal Medicine Residency Program, Associate Professor of Internal Medicine, and a hospitalist at the University of Michigan. She has received teaching awards at the University of Michigan from both medical students and residents, including the Marvin Pollard Award for Outstanding Teaching of Residents, Richard D. Judge Award for Outstanding Teaching of Medical Students, Kaiser Permanente Award for Excellence in Clinical Teaching, and the Graduate Medical Education Mentor of the Year Award.

Dr. Hartley received her medical degree from Wayne State University School of Medicine, where she also served as a resident and chief medical resident.

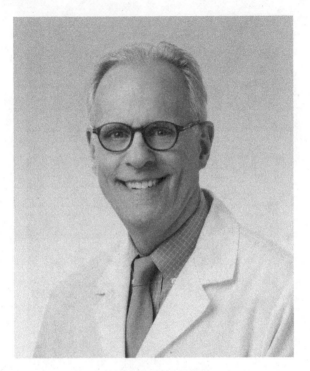

Robert Hirschtick, MD

Robert Hirschtick, MD, is Associate Professor Emeritus of Medicine at the Feinberg School of Medicine, Northwestern University. He served as medicine clerkship site director at Chicago's Jesse Brown VA Medical Center for 25 years. He has won numerous teaching awards including the Outstanding Clinical Teacher Award, the Robert J. Winter Clinical Teacher Award, the George Joost Award for Outstanding Clinical Teacher, and the "Teaching Hall of Fame" Award. He is a frequent contributor to "A Piece of My Mind" in the *Journal of the American Medical Association*.

Dr. Hirschtick received his medical degree from the University of Illinois College of Medicine and did his residency at Evanston Hospital/Northwestern.

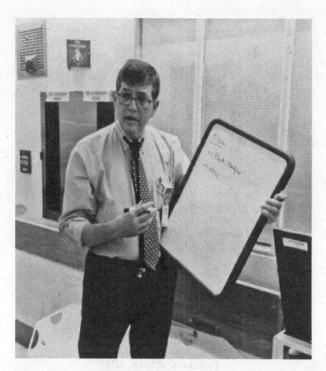

Daniel Hunt, MD, FACP

Daniel P. Hunt, MD, FACP, is Division Director of Hospital Medicine and Professor of Medicine at Emory University. He has been awarded more than 35 major teaching awards, including the Alfred Kranes Award for Excellence in Clinical Teaching from Massachusetts General Hospital, Best Clinical Instructor Award from Harvard Medical School, and the Society of Hospital Medicine's Award for Excellence in Teaching. Dr. Hunt has been the primary discussant for six "Clinicopathologic Case Conferences" published in the *New England Journal of Medicine* and has served as the unknown case discussant at national conferences.

Dr. Hunt received his medical degree from Vanderbilt University School and completed his internal medicine residency at Vanderbilt, with his third year at Baylor College of Medicine.

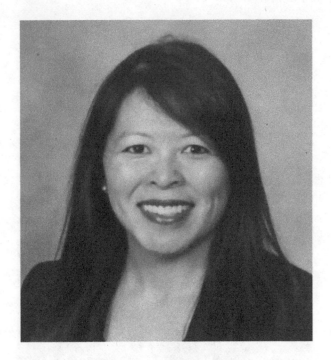

Deanne Kashiwagi, MD

Deanne Kashiwagi, MD, is Deputy Chief Medical Officer of Sheikh Shakhbout Medical City (SSMC), a joint venture with Mayo Clinic, and Program Director of the Internal Medicine Residency Program at SSMC. She previously served as Vice Chair of Hospital Internal Medicine at Mayo Clinic. She has received several teaching awards, including Excellence in Clinical Teaching at the Mayo School of Graduate Medical Education (2018, 2019) and Teacher of the Year–Hall of Fame (2019, 2020).

   Dr. Kashiwagi received her medical degree from Loyola University of Chicago Stritch School of Medicine and completed her residency at Indiana University School of Medicine.

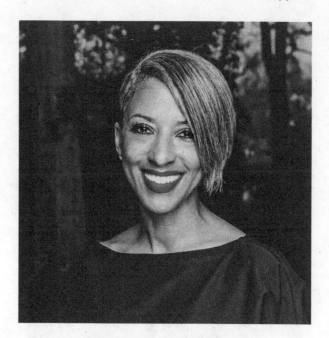

Kimberly Manning, MD

Kimberly Manning, MD, is Professor of Medicine and Associate Chair of Diversity, Equity, and Inclusion at Emory University School of Medicine in Atlanta, Georgia. She has won numerous teaching awards, including the ACGME Parker J. Palmer Courage to Teach Award, the Evangeline Papageorge Distinguished Teaching Award, and the Juha P. Kokko Teaching Award for Best Overall Teacher (2011, 2013). Her blog "Reflections of a Grady Doctor" was named in the top four medical blogs by "O" magazine.

Dr. Manning received her medical degree from Meharry Medical College and completed a combined internal medicine and pediatrics residency, as well as a chief residency, at Case Western Reserve University/MetroHealth.

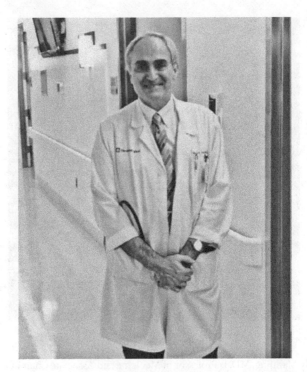

Robert Mayock, MD

Robert Mayock, MD, is an attending physician for inpatient medicine teaching services at the Cleveland Clinic. He has won numerous teaching awards including being a seven-time recipient of the Cleveland Clinic Department of Medicine Teacher of the Year award. This award has since been renamed in his honor, titled the "Robert Mayock Teaching Award." He is also a recipient of the Bruce Hubbard Stewart Fellowship Award for his humanistic approach to the practice of medicine.

Dr. Mayock received his medical degree from Case Western Reserve University and completed his residency at the Indiana University Medical Center.

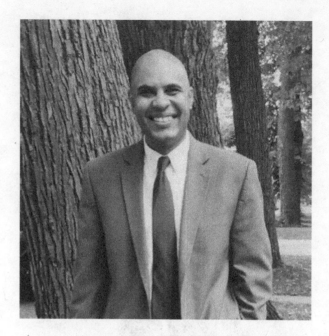

Benjamin Mba, MBBS, MRCP (UK)

Benjamin Mba, MBBS, MRCP (UK), is Professor of Internal Medicine at Rush University Medical Center, Associate Chair of Medicine for Faculty Development, and Associate Program Director of the Internal Medicine Residency Program at the John H. Stroger, Jr. Hospital of Cook County Chicago (former Cook County Hospital). Dr. Mba is a four-time recipient of the Sir William Osler Award for teaching of internal medicine from the Department of Medicine at Stroger Hospital, a four-time recipient of the Division of Hospital Medicine's Cooker Award for in-patient medicine teaching and team leadership, and a three-time recipient of the Department of Medicine Excellence in Medical Student Education Award. He has received a Certificate of Appreciation from the American College of Physicians (ACP) for mentoring.

Dr. Mba graduated from medical school in Nigeria. He initially completed an internal medicine residency training program in the United Kingdom before relocating to the United States. He completed a second medicine residency program at the Cook County Hospital in Chicago, where he also served as a chief medical resident.

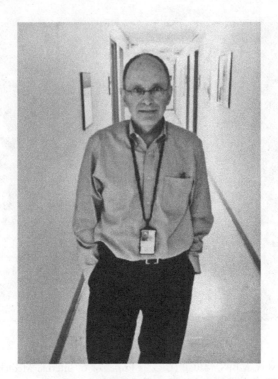

Steven McGee, MD

Steven McGee, MD, is Professor Emeritus of Medicine at the University of Washington in Seattle where he served as a Staff Physician at the Seattle VA Medical Center. He has received numerous teaching awards, including the Marvin Turck Outstanding Teaching Award, Teacher Superior in Perpetuity Award, the Margaret Anderson Award, two Attending-of-the-Year Awards, the Paul Beeson Teaching Award, and the National Alpha Omega Alpha Distinguished Teacher Award. He has published extensively on bedside rounding and evidence-based diagnosis, including the highly acclaimed book *Evidence-Based Physical Diagnosis*.

Dr. McGee is a graduate of Washington University School of Medicine in St. Louis, and he completed his internship, residency, chief residency, and fellowship in infectious diseases at the University of Washington School of Medicine in Seattle.

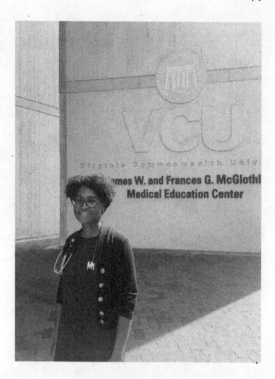

Georgia McIntosh, MD

Georgia McIntosh, MD, is Associate Professor in the Division of Hospital Medicine and Associate Chair of Quality and Safety for the Department of Internal Medicine at Virginia Commonwealth University Health. She has received several teaching awards, including Outstanding Ward Attending, the Dr. J. David Markham Award for Excellence in Teaching, and the Leonard Tow Humanism in Medicine Award presented by the Arnold P. Gold Foundation. Dr. McIntosh was voted a 2020 "Top Doc" by her peers in *Richmond Magazine*.

Dr. McIntosh received her medical degree from Pennsylvania State University College of Medicine and completed her internal medicine and chief residency at Virginia Commonwealth University.

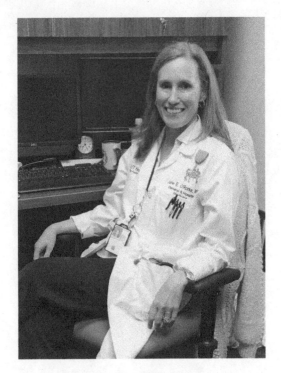

Jane O'Rorke, MD, FACP

Jane O'Rorke, MD, FACP, is Professor of Medicine in the Division of Hospital Medicine and Program Director for the Internal Medicine Residency at the University of Texas Health Science Center, San Antonio. She has won numerous teaching awards, including Southern Society of General Internal Medicine Clinician Educator-of-the-Year, Outstanding Teacher-of-the-Year Award for the Division of General Internal Medicine, Division of Hospital Medicine Hospitalist Teaching Award, and the University of Texas Presidential Teaching Excellence Award.

Dr. O'Rorke received her medical degree from the State University of New York Health Science Center and completed her internal medicine and chief residency at the University of Texas Health Science Center. She completed a Faculty Development Fellowship at the University of North Carolina, Chapel Hill.

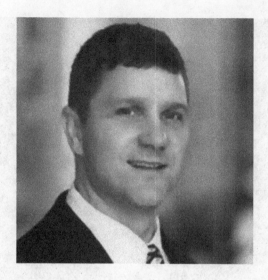

E. Lee Poythress, MD

E. Lee Poythress, MD, is Associate Dean of Student Affairs, Associate Professor of Medicine, and Director of the Ben Taub Hospital Wound Care Clinic at Baylor College of Medicine in Houston. He has won numerous teaching awards, including being a seven-time recipient of the Department of Internal Medicine Outstanding Faculty Educator Award and three-time recipient of the Baylor College of Medicine Medical School Outstanding Faculty Award. In 2016, he was inducted into the Baylor College of Medicine Medical School "Teaching Hall of Fame."

Dr. Poythress received his medical degree from the University of Virginia Medical School. He completed an internal medicine residency and geriatrics fellowship at the Baylor College of Medicine.

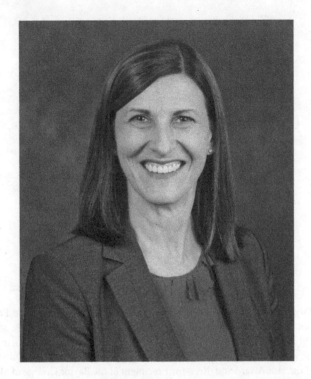

Christine Seibert, MD, MACP

Christine Seibert, MD, MACP, is Associate Dean for Medical Student Education and Services at the University of Wisconsin School of Medicine and Public Health, as well as a Professor of Medicine. She was the recipient of the UW-Madison Chancellor's Hilldale Award for Excellence in Teaching and the School of Medicine and Public Health's Dean's Teaching Award. She has also been elected a fellow in the University of Wisconsin Teaching Academy. Dr. Seibert practices primary care general internal medicine in addition to her ward attending duties.

Dr. Seibert received her medical degree from Northwestern University. She completed an internship and residency in internal medicine at Brigham and Women's Hospital in Boston.

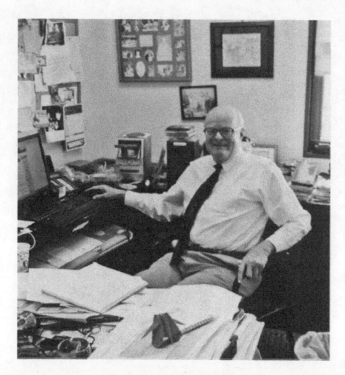

Lawrence M. Tierney Jr., MD

Lawrence M. Tierney, Jr., MD, is Professor Emeritus of Medicine at the University of California at San Francisco (UCSF) School of Medicine where he served as the Associate Chief of Medicine at the San Francisco VA Medical Center for several decades. He received countless teaching awards, including the Kaiser Award and the UCSF Distinction in Teaching Award. He has been a visiting professor at more than 100 institutions around the world and is widely hailed as a master diagnostician.

Dr. Tierney—aka "LT"—received his medical degree from the University of Maryland School of Medicine. He did his residency training at both Emory and UCSF, and he completed a chief residency at UCSF.

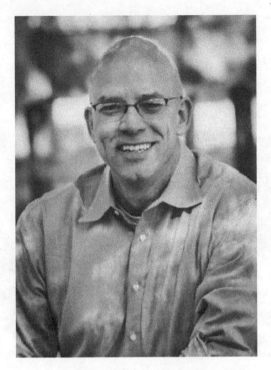

Jeff Wiese, MD, MACP, MHM

Jeff Wiese, MD, MACP, MHM, is a Professor of Medicine. He has previously served as Chief of the Charity Medical Service, the Director of the Tulane Internal Medicine Residency Program, and the Senior Associate Dean for Graduate Medical Education at the Tulane University Health Sciences Center. He has won more than 50 teaching awards, including being a six-time winner of Tulane's Attending of the Year Award. His other awards include the Society of Hospital Medicine's Education Award, the Accreditation Council for Graduate Medical Education (ACGME)'s Parker Palmer Courage to Teach Award, the Association of American Medical Colleges (AAMC)'s Robert J. Glaser Distinguished Teacher Award, the American College of Physicians (ACP)'s Walter J. McDonald Award, and the Society of General Internal Medicine's Mid-Career Mentorship Award. He is the author of the book *Teaching in the Hospital*.

Dr. Wiese received his medical degree from Johns Hopkins School of Medicine and completed his internal medicine residency, chief residency, and a medical education fellowship at the University of California at San Francisco.

References

Chapter 1: Teaching Medicine

1. 2021 FACTS: Enrollment, graduates, and MD-PhD data. Table 1: Applicants, matriculants, enrollment, and graduates of U.S. medical schools, 2012–2013 through 2021–2022. Association of American Medical Colleges, 2021. (Accessed May 6, 2022, at https://www.aamc.org/media/37816/download?attachment.)
2. American Hospital Association. Teaching hospitals. (Accessed May 6, 2022, at https://www.aha.org/advocacy/teaching-hospitals.)
3. Fisher K. Academic health centers save millions of lives. Association of American Medical Colleges, 2019. (Accessed May 6, 2022, at https://www.aamc.org/news-insights/academic-health-centers-save-millions-lives.)
4. Whitt N, Harvey R, McLeod G, Child S. How many health professionals does a patient see during an average hospital stay? N Z Med J 2007;120:U2517.
5. Doyle C, Lennox L, Bell D. A systematic review of evidence on the links between patient experience and clinical safety and effectiveness. BMJ Open 2013;3.
6. Fact Sheet: FDA at a glance. U.S. Food & Drug Administration, 2020. (Accessed May 10, 2022, at https://www.fda.gov/about-fda/fda-basics/fact-sheet-fda-glance.)
7. Accreditation Council for Graduate Medical Education. ACGME Common Program Requirements section VI with background and intent. 2017. (Accessed May 24, 2022, at https://www.acgme.org/globalassets/PFAssets/ProgramRequirements/CPRs_Section-VI_with-Background-and-Intent_2017-01.pdf.)
8. Freudenberger HJ. Staff burn-out. J Soc Issues 1974;30:159–65.
9. Rothenberger DA. Physician burnout and well-being: A systematic review and framework for action. Dis Colon Rectum 2017;60:567–76.
10. Rotenstein LS, Torre M, Ramos MA, et al. Prevalence of burnout among physicians: A systematic review. JAMA 2018;320:1131–50.
11. Dewa CS, Loong D, Bonato S, Trojanowski L. The relationship between physician burnout and quality of healthcare in terms of safety and acceptability: A systematic review. BMJ Open 2017;7:e015141.
12. Dewa CS, Loong D, Bonato S, Trojanowski L, Rea M. The relationship between resident burnout and safety-related and acceptability-related quality of healthcare: A systematic literature review. BMC Med Educ 2017;17:195.

13. Hall LH, Johnson J, Watt I, Tsipa A, O'Connor DB. Healthcare staff wellbeing, burnout, and patient safety: A systematic review. PLoS One 2016;11:e0159015.

14. Cochran A, Hauschild T, Elder WB, Neumayer LA, Brasel KJ, Crandall ML. Perceived gender-based barriers to careers in academic surgery. Am J Surg 2013;206:263–8.

15. Adesoye T, Mangurian C, Choo EK, et al. Perceived discrimination experienced by physician mothers and desired workplace changes: A cross-sectional survey. JAMA Intern Med 2017;177:1033–6.

16. Hu YY, Ellis RJ, Hewitt DB, et al. Discrimination, abuse, harassment, and burnout in surgical residency training. N Engl J Med 2019;381:1741–52.

17. Chetty R, Stepner M, Abraham S, et al. The association between income and life expectancy in the United States, 2001–2014. JAMA 2016;315:1750–66.

18. Castiglioni A, Shewchuk RM, Willett LL, Heudebert GR, Centor RM. A pilot study using nominal group technique to assess residents' perceptions of successful attending rounds. J Gen Intern Med 2008;23:1060–5.

19. Elnicki DM, Cooper A. Medical students' perceptions of the elements of effective inpatient teaching by attending physicians and housestaff. J Gen Intern Med 2005;20:635–9.

20. Mann KV. Theoretical perspectives in medical education: Past experience and future possibilities. Med Educ 2011;45:60–8.

21. Houchens N, Quinn M, Harrod M, Cronin DT, Hartley S, Saint S. Strategies of female teaching attending physicians to navigate gender-based challenges: An exploratory qualitative study. J Hosp Med 2020;15:454–60.

22. Houchens N, Harrod M, Moody S, Fowler K, Saint S. Techniques and behaviors associated with exemplary inpatient general medicine teaching: An exploratory qualitative study. J Hosp Med 2017;12:503–9.

Chapter 2: Unique Individuals, Shared Qualities

1. Wachter RM, Goldman L. The emerging role of "hospitalists" in the American health care system. N Engl J Med 1996;335:514–17.

2. Wood D. 15 surprising facts about hospitalists. Staff Care, 2020. (Accessed May 11, 2022, at https://www.staffcare.com/physician-blogs/15-surprising-facts-about-hospitalists-in-2020/.)

3. Wachter RM, Goldman L. Zero to 50,000: The 20th anniversary of the hospitalist. N Engl J Med 2016;375:1009–11.

4. American Hospital Association. Creating the hospital of the future: The implications for hospital-focused physician practice. 2012. (Accessed May 11, 2022, at https://www.aha.org/ahahret-guides/2012-11-01-creating-hospital-future-implications-hospital-focused-physician-practice.)

5. Harkin B, Webb TL, Chang BP, et al. Does monitoring goal progress promote goal attainment? A meta-analysis of the experimental evidence. Psychol Bull 2016;142:198–229.

Chapter 3: Underrepresented Voices

1. Association of American Medical Colleges. Underrepresented in medicine definition. (Accessed May 9, 2022, at https://www.aamc.org/what-we-do/equ ity-diversity-inclusion/underrepresented-in-medicine.)
2. Komaromy M, Bindman AB, Haber RJ, Sande MA. Sexual harassment in medical training. N Engl J Med 1993;328:322–6.
3. Cochran A, Hauschild T, Elder WB, Neumayer LA, Brasel KJ, Crandall ML. Perceived gender-based barriers to careers in academic surgery. Am J Surg 2013;206:263–8.
4. Choo EK, van Dis J, Kass D. Time's up for medicine? Only time will tell. N Engl J Med 2018;379:1592–3.
5. Adesoye T, Mangurian C, Choo EK, et al. Perceived discrimination experienced by physician mothers and desired workplace changes: A cross-sectional survey. JAMA Intern Med 2017;177:1033–6.
6. More ES. Restoring the Balance: Women Physicians and the Profession of Medicine, 1850–1995. Cambridge, MA: Harvard University Press; 2001.
7. Houchens N, Quinn M, Harrod M, Cronin DT, Hartley S, Saint S. Strategies of female teaching attending physicians to navigate gender-based challenges: An exploratory qualitative study. J Hosp Med 2020;15:454–60.
8. 2021 FACTS. Applicants and matriculants data. Table A-7.2: Applicants, first-time applicants, acceptees, and matriculants to U.S. medical schools by sex, 2012–2013 through 2021–2022. Association of American Medical Colleges, 2021. (Accessed May 24, 2022, at https://www.aamc.org/system/files/2021-11/2021_FACTS_Tabl e_A-7.2.pdf.)
9. U.S. Medical School Faculty. Table 13: U.S. medical school faculty by gender, rank, and department. Association of American Medical Colleges, 2021. (Accessed May 10, 2022, at https://www.aamc.org/media/9736/download?att achment.)
10. Heilman ME. Description and prescription: How gender stereotypes prevent women's ascent up the organizational ladder. J Soc Issues 2001;57:657–74.
11. Fnais N, Soobiah C, Chen MH, et al. Harassment and discrimination in medical training: A systematic review and meta-analysis. Acad Med 2014;89:817–27.
12. Sandoval RS, Afolabi T, Said J, Dunleavy S, Chatterjee A, Olveczky D. Building a tool kit for medical and dental students: Addressing microaggressions and discrimination on the wards. MedEdPORTAL 2020;16:10893.
13. Hu YY, Ellis RJ, Hewitt DB, et al. Discrimination, abuse, harassment, and burnout in surgical residency training. N Engl J Med 2019;381:1741–52.
14. Vargas EA, Brassel ST, Cortina LM, Settles IH, Johnson TRB, Jagsi R. #MedToo: A large-scale examination of the incidence and impact of sexual harassment of physicians and other faculty at an academic medical center. J Womens Health (Larchmt) 2020;29:13–20.
15. Chopra V, Saint S, Vaughn V. The Mentoring Guide: Helping Mentors and Mentees Succeed. Ann Arbor, MI: Michigan Publishing Services; 2019.
16. Epictetus Quotes. Goodreads. (Accessed May 11, 2022, at https://www.goodre ads.com/quotes/7588248-we-cannot-choose-our-external-circumstances-but-we-can-always.)

17. Lorde A. Sister Outsider: Essays and Speeches. Trumansburg, NY: Crossing Press; 2007.

Chapter 4: Building the Team

1. Ludmerer KM. Time to Heal: American Medical Education from the Turn of the Century to the Era of Managed Care. New York, NY: Oxford University Press; 1999.
2. Saint S. Caring for veterans: A privilege and a duty. The Conversation, 2016. (Accessed May 11, 2022, at https://theconversation.com/caring-for-veterans-a-privilege-and-a-duty-67823.)
3. Ramani S. Twelve tips to improve bedside teaching. Med Teach 2003;25:112–15.
4. Bain K. What the Best College Teachers Do. Cambridge, MA: Harvard University Press; 2011.
5. Goebel EA, Cristancho SM, Driman DK. Pimping in residency: The emotional roller-coaster of a pedagogical method: A qualitative study using interviews and rich picture drawings. Teach Learn Med 2019;31:497–505.
6. Kendra T. Bo Schembechler's legendary "The Team" speech still rings true today in high school football. 2011. (Accessed May 11, 2022, at https://www.mlive.com/sports/muskegon/2011/08/bo_schembechlers_legendary_the.html.)
7. Baker DP, Day R, Salas E. Teamwork as an essential component of high-reliability organizations. Health Serv Res 2006;41:1576–98.
8. Wenger E. How We Learn. Communities of practice: The social fabric of a learning organization. Healthc Forum J 1996;39:20–6.
9. Page SE. The Diversity Bonus: How Great Teams Pay Off in the Knowledge Economy. Princeton, NJ: Princeton University Press; 2017.
10. Mann KV. Theoretical perspectives in medical education: Past experience and future possibilities. Med Educ 2011;45:60–8.
11. Weinstein D. Ensuring an effective physician workforce for the United States: Recommendations for graduate medical education to meet the needs of the public. Content and format of GME (2nd of two conferences). May 2011; Atlanta, GA.
12. Cribb A, Bignold S. Towards the reflexive medical school: The hidden curriculum and medical education research. Stud High Educ 1999;24:195–209.
13. Sutcliffe KM, Lewton E, Rosenthal MM. Communication failures: An insidious contributor to medical mishaps. Acad Med 2004;79:186–94.
14. Karliner LS, Jacobs EA, Chen AH, Mutha S. Do professional interpreters improve clinical care for patients with limited English proficiency? A systematic review of the literature. Health Serv Res 2007;42:727–54.
15. Dames S, Tonnerre C, Saint S, Jones SR. Clinical problem-solving: Don't know much about history. N Engl J Med 2005;352:2338–42.

Chapter 5: A Safe, Supportive Environment

1. Mann KV. Theoretical perspectives in medical education: Past experience and future possibilities. Med Educ 2011;45:60–8.
2. Sutkin G, Wagner E, Harris I, Schiffer R. What makes a good clinical teacher in medicine? A review of the literature. Acad Med 2008;83:452–66.
3. Chopra V, Saint S. "The tunnel at the end of the light": Preparing to attend on the inpatient medical wards. JAMA 2017;318:1007–8.
4. Strohbehn GW, Jaffe T, Houchens N. Sketching an approach to clinical education: What we can learn from improvisation. J Grad Med Educ 2020;12:388–91.
5. Saint S, Chopra V. Thirty Rules for Healthcare Leaders. Ann Arbor, MI: Michigan Publishing Services; 2019.
6. Goleman D. Emotional Intelligence: Why It Can Matter More Than IQ. 10th Anniversary ed. New York, NY: Random House; 2005.

Chapter 6: Bedside and Beyond

1. Shankel SW, Mazzaferri EL. Teaching the resident in internal medicine: Present practices and suggestions for the future. JAMA 1986;256:725–9.
2. Block L, Habicht R, Wu AW, et al. In the wake of the 2003 and 2011 duty hours regulations, how do internal medicine interns spend their time? J Gen Intern Med 2013;28:1042–7.
3. Society of Bedside Medicine. Creating Human Connection. (Accessed May 12, 2022, at https://bedsidemedicine.org/.)
4. Accreditation Council for Graduate Medical Education. Back to bedside. (Accessed May 12, 2022, at https://www.acgme.org/residents-and-fellows/back-to-bedside/.)
5. Appold B, Saint S, Gupta A. Comparing Oral Case Presentation Formats on Rounds: A Survey Study. SHM Converge; 2022.
6. Clinical Skills Education LLC. Easy auscultation. (Accessed May 12, 2022, at https://www.easyauscultation.com/egophony.)
7. Gladstone DJ, Spring M, Dorian P, et al. Atrial fibrillation in patients with cryptogenic stroke. N Engl J Med 2014;370:2467–77.
8. Saint S, Chopra V. The Saint-Chopra Guide to Inpatient Medicine. 4th ed. New York, NY: Oxford University Press; 2018.

Chapter 7: How to Think About Thinking

1. Eva KW. What every teacher needs to know about clinical reasoning. Med Educ 2005;39:98–106.
2. Irby DM. Excellence in clinical teaching: Knowledge transformation and development required. Med Educ 2014;48:776–84.

3. Centor RM, Willett LL. Becoming a better ward attending: Two experts discuss 10 modifiable behaviors. ACP Hospitalist, 2008. (Accessed May 13, 2022, at https://acphospitalist.acponline.org/archives/2008/05/attending.htm.)
4. Bain K. What the Best College Teachers Do. Cambridge, MA: Harvard University Press; 2011.
5. Maxwell M. Introduction to the Socratic method and its effect on critical thinking. 2009–2019. (Accessed May 13, 2022, at http://www.socraticmethod.net.)
6. The Clinical Problem Solvers. (Accessed May 13, 2022, at https://clinicalproblemsolving.com/.)

Chapter 8: Role Models

1. Wright S, Wong A, Newill C. The impact of role models on medical students. J Gen Intern Med 1997;12:53–6.
2. Harkin B, Webb TL, Chang BP, et al. Does monitoring goal progress promote goal attainment? A meta-analysis of the experimental evidence. Psychol Bull 2016;142:198–229.
3. Branch WT, Jr., Kern D, Haidet P, et al. Teaching the human dimensions of care in clinical settings. JAMA 2001;286:1067–74.
4. Neumann M, Edelhauser F, Tauschel D, et al. Empathy decline and its reasons: A systematic review of studies with medical students and residents. Acad Med 2011;86:996–1009.
5. Medical School Objectives Project. Report I: Learning Objectives for Medical Student Education. Guidelines for Medical Schools. Washington, DC: Association of American Medical Colleges; 1998.
6. Detsky AS, Verma AA. A new model for medical education: Celebrating restraint. JAMA 2012;308:1329–30.

Chapter 9: Mentors and Sponsors

1. West M, Armit K, Loewenthal L, Eckert R, West T, Lee A. Leadership and Leadership Development in Healthcare: The Evidence Base. London: The Faculty of Medical Leadership and Management; 2015.
2. Clemmer TP, Spuhler VJ, Oniki TA, Horn SD. Results of a collaborative quality improvement program on outcomes and costs in a tertiary critical care unit. Crit Care Med 1999;27:1768–74.
3. Wong CA, Cummings GG. The relationship between nursing leadership and patient outcomes: A systematic review. J Nurs Manag 2007;15:508–21.
4. Squires M, Tourangeau A, Spence Laschinger HK, Doran D. The link between leadership and safety outcomes in hospitals. J Nurs Manag 2010;18:914–25.
5. Weberg D. Transformational leadership and staff retention: An evidence review with implications for healthcare systems. Nurs Adm Q 2010;34:246–58.

6. Curry LA, Spatz E, Cherlin E, et al. What distinguishes top-performing hospitals in acute myocardial infarction mortality rates? A qualitative study. Ann Intern Med 2011;154:384–90.

7. Commission on Patient Safety and Quality Assurance. Building a Culture of Patient Safety: Report of the Commission on Patient Safety and Quality Assurance. Dublin: Department of Health & Children; 2008.

8. Shanafelt TD, Gorringe G, Menaker R, et al. Impact of organizational leadership on physician burnout and satisfaction. Mayo Clin Proc 2015;90:432–40.

9. Cummings GG, Tate K, Lee S, et al. Leadership styles and outcome patterns for the nursing workforce and work environment: A systematic review. Int J Nurs Stud 2018;85:19–60.

10. Hartmann CW, Meterko M, Rosen AK, et al. Relationship of hospital organizational culture to patient safety climate in the Veterans Health Administration. Med Care Res Rev 2009;66:320–38.

11. Goleman D, Boyatzis R, McKee A. The New Leaders: Transforming the Art of Leadership. London: Time Warner; 2003.

12. Chopra V, Arora VM, Saint S. Will you be my mentor? Four archetypes to help mentees succeed in academic medicine. JAMA Intern Med 2018;178:175–6.

13. O'Donnell BRJ. The Odyssey's millenia-old model of mentorship. The Atlantic Monthly Group, 2017. (Accessed May 24, 2022, at https://www.theatlantic.com/business/archive/2017/10/the-odyssey-mentorship/542676/.)

14. Foust-Cummings H, Dinolfo S, Kohler J. Sponsoring Women to Success. New York, NY: Catalyst; 2011.

15. Pearce CL, Sims HP. Vertical versus shared leadership as predictors of the effectiveness of change management teams: An examination of aversive, directive, transactional, transformational, and empowering leader behaviors. Group Dyn Theory Res Pract 2002;6:172–97.

16. Ensley MD, Hmieleski KM, Pearce CL. The importance of vertical and shared leadership within new venture top management teams: Implications for the performance of startups. Leadersh Q 2006;17:217–31.

17. Orman S. I didn't become a mentor to make others more like me. Linkedin 2015. (Accessed May 24, 2022, at https://www.linkedin.com/pulse/mentor-who-shaped-me-i-didnt-become-make-others-more-like-suze-orman.)

18. Moniz MH, Saint S. Leadership & professional development: Be the change you want to see. J Hosp Med 2019;14:254.

19. LAPD Motto. LAPD Online. (Accessed May 18, 2022, at https://www.lapdonline.org/lapd-motto/.)

20. Saint S, Chopra V. How doctors can be better mentors. Harv Bus Rev 2018. https://hbr.org/2018/10/how-doctors-can-be-better-mentors.

21. Chopra V, Edelson DP, Saint S. Mentorship malpractice. JAMA 2016;315:1453–4.

22. Chopra V, Saint S. Mindful mentorship. Healthc 2020;8:100390.

23. Waljee JF, Chopra V, Saint S. Mentoring millennials. JAMA 2018;319:1547–8.

24. Borges NJ, Manuel RS, Elam CL, Jones BJ. Differences in motives between Millennial and Generation X medical students. Med Educ 2010;44:570–6.
25. Sutkin G, Wagner E, Harris I, Schiffer R. What makes a good clinical teacher in medicine? A review of the literature. Acad Med 2008;83:452–66.
26. Houchens N, Sivils SL, Koester E, Ratz D, Ridenour J, Saint S. Fueling leadership in yourself: A leadership development program for all types of health-care workers. Leadersh Health Serv 2021;34:98–111.
27. Chopra V, Woods MD, Saint S. The four golden rules of effective menteeship. BMJ 2016;354:i4147.

Chapter 10: The Stories We Share

1. Heisler M, Bouknight RR, Hayward RA, Smith DM, Kerr EA. The relative importance of physician communication, participatory decision making, and patient understanding in diabetes self-management. J Gen Intern Med 2002;17:243–52.
2. Hojat M, Louis DZ, Markham FW, Wender R, Rabinowitz C, Gonnella JS. Physicians' empathy and clinical outcomes for diabetic patients. Acad Med 2011;86:359–64.
3. Ong LML, de Haes JCJM, Hoos AM, Lammes FB. Doctor–patient communication: A review of the literature. Soc Sci Med 1995;40:903–18.
4. Safran DG, Taira DA, Rogers WH, Kosinski M, Ware JE, Tarlov AR. Linking primary care performance to outcomes of care. J Fam Pract 1998;47:213–20.
5. Renzi C, Abeni D, Picardi A, et al. Factors associated with patient satisfaction with care among dermatological outpatients. Br J Dermatol 2001;145:617–23.
6. Stewart M, Brown JB, Donner A, et al. The impact of patient-centered care on outcomes. J Fam Pract 2000;49:796–804.
7. Ambady N, Laplante D, Nguyen T, Rosenthal R, Chaumeton N, Levinson W. Surgeons' tone of voice: A clue to malpractice history. Surgery 2002;132:5–9.
8. Marvel MK, Epstein RM, Flowers K, Beckman HB. Soliciting the patient's agenda: Have we improved? JAMA 1999;281:283–7.
9. Mauksch LB, Dugdale DC, Dodson S, Epstein R. Relationship, communication, and efficiency in the medical encounter: Creating a clinical model from a literature review. Arch Intern Med 2008;168:1387–95.
10. Tulsky JA. Interventions to enhance communication among patients, providers, and families. J Palliat Med 2005;8(Suppl 1):S95–102.
11. Norgaard B, Ammentorp J, Ohm Kyvik K, Kofoed PE. Communication skills training increases self-efficacy of health care professionals. J Contin Educ Health Prof 2012;32:90–7.
12. Weng HC, Hung CM, Liu YT, et al. Associations between emotional intelligence and doctor burnout, job satisfaction and patient satisfaction. Med Educ 2011;45:835–42.

13. Jensen FB, Gulbrandsen P, Dahl FA, Krupat E, Frankel RM, Finset A. Effectiveness of a short course in clinical communication skills for hospital doctors: Results of a crossover randomized controlled trial (ISRCTN22153332). Patient Educ Couns 2011;84:163–9.
14. Boissy A, Windover AK, Bokar D, et al. Communication skills training for physicians improves patient satisfaction. J Gen Intern Med 2016;31:755–61.
15. Makoul G. Essential elements of communication in medical encounters: The Kalamazoo Consensus Statement. Acad Med 2001;76:390–3.
16. Wolpaw DR, Shapiro D. The virtues of irrelevance. N Engl J Med 2014;370:1283–5.
17. Safder T. The name of the dog. N Engl J Med 2018;379:1299–301.
18. Petrilli CM, Mack M, Petrilli JJ, Hickner A, Saint S, Chopra V. Understanding the role of physician attire on patient perceptions: A systematic review of the literature: Targeting Attire to Improve Likelihood of Rapport (TAILOR) investigators. BMJ Open 2015;5:e006578.
19. Petrilli CM, Saint S, Jennings JJ, et al. Understanding patient preference for physician attire: A cross-sectional observational study of 10 academic medical centres in the USA. BMJ Open 2018;8:e021239.
20. Neumann M, Edelhauser F, Tauschel D, et al. Empathy decline and its reasons: A systematic review of studies with medical students and residents. Acad Med 2011;86:996–1009.
21. Pargament KI, Mahoney A. Theory: Sacred matters: Sanctification as a vital topic for the psychology of religion. Int J Psychol Relig 2005;15:179–98.
22. Lomax JW, Kripal JJ, Pargament KI. Perspectives on "sacred moments" in psychotherapy. Am J Psychiatry 2011;168:12–18.
23. Radetsky M. Sudden intimacies. JAMA 1985;254.
24. Zulman DM, Haverfield MC, Shaw JG, et al. Practices to foster physician presence and connection with patients in the clinical encounter. JAMA 2020;323:70–81.

Chapter 11: The Sacred Act of Healing

1. Institute of Medicine, Committee on Quality of Health Care in America. Crossing the Quality Chasm: A New Health System for the 21st Century. Washington, DC: National Academies Press; 2001.
2. Hojat M, Louis DZ, Markham FW, Wender R, Rabinowitz C, Gonnella JS. Physicians' empathy and clinical outcomes for diabetic patients. Acad Med 2011;86:359–64.
3. Ong LML, de Haes JCJM, Hoos AM, Lammes FB. Doctor-patient communication: A review of the literature. Soc Sci Med 1995;40:903–18.
4. Peabody FW. The care of the patient. JAMA 1927;88:877–82.
5. Misra-Hebert AD, Isaacson JH. Overcoming health care disparities via better cross-cultural communication and health literacy. Cleve Clin J Med 2012;79:127–33.

Chapter 12: Caring During Crisis

1. Kahn MW. Etiquette-based medicine. N Engl J Med 2008;358:1988–9.
2. Wright S, Wong A, Newill C. The impact of role models on medical students. J Gen Intern Med 1997;12:53–6.
3. Swayden KJ, Anderson KK, Connelly LM, Moran JS, McMahon JK, Arnold PM. Effect of sitting vs. standing on perception of provider time at bedside: A pilot study. Patient Educ Couns 2012;86:166–71.
4. Houchens N, Tipirneni R. Compassionate communication amid the COVID-19 pandemic. J Hosp Med 2020;15:437–9.

Index

For the benefit of digital users, indexed terms that span two pages (e.g., 52–53) may, on occasion, appear on only one of those pages.

Figures and boxes are indicated by *f* and *b* following the page number